"An extremely moving, personal and amazing journey told in a clear, honest and inspiring manner. This book will definitely help not only patients, their family members and friends, but also health care professionals."

—Eric S. Freedland, M.D.
Diabetes researcher and columnist for diabetesincontrol.com

"As a diabetes nurse educator, it has been a pleasure for me to work with and get to know the Plunkett family. In this book, they honestly and openly share their journey through the first few years of life with diabetes. They beautifully illustrate that when a child has diabetes, it affects everyone in the family, not just the child. When I see newly diagnosed families for their first outpatient visit, often they are doing quite well with the tasks of diabetes—the injections, the blood sugar checks, the meal planning, but the largest challenge that they are facing is the emotional one. This book addresses the effects of chronic illness on the whole family, and it will help others realize they are not alone in their feelings."

—Kristen Rice, R.N., B.S.N., C.D.E.
Diabetes Nurse Educator
Children's Hospital Boston

"The book was wonderful! The story illustrates how daunting, but also crucial, dietary changes can be."

—Jan Hangen, M.S., R.D., L.D.N.
Clinical Nutrition Specialist
Children's Hospital Boston

The Challenge of
Childhood Diabetes

The Challenge of Childhood Diabetes

Family Strategies for Raising a Healthy Child

Includes a Survival Guide for Parents

By Laura Plunkett
with Linda Weltner

iUniverse, Inc.
New York Lincoln Shanghai

The Challenge of Childhood Diabetes
Family Strategies for Raising a Healthy Child

iUniverse books may be ordered through booksellers or by contacting:

iUniverse
2021 Pine Lake Road, Suite 100
Lincoln, NE 68512
www.iuniverse.com
1-800-Authors (1-800-288-4677)

The information, ideas and suggestions in this book are not intended as a substitute for professional medical advice. Before following any suggestions contained in this book, you should first consult your personal physician.

Neither the author nor the publisher shall be liable or responsible for any loss or damage allegedly arising as a consequence of your use or application of any information or suggestions in this book.

ISBN-13: 978-0-595-38625-3 (pbk)
ISBN-13: 978-0-595-83005-3 (ebk)
ISBN-10: 0-595-38625-3 (pbk)
ISBN-10: 0-595-83005-6 (ebk)

Printed in the United States of America

Our family offers this book as an invitation

—One we wish we'd had from the beginning—

To face this challenge with focus and intensity,

To meet the future one day at a time,

To follow your instincts,

And to be committed to keeping

the love between you alive.

May you be kind to yourself along the way.

I dedicate this book to my parents,

Linda and Jack Weltner,

who show up,

tell the truth,

live with integrity,

and hold us all

with an extraordinary amount

of love and commitment.

And with love to

Annie Bell

(1948-2004)

for friendship and courage.

Contents

▼

Foreword by Dr. Ann Wyttenbach.. xv

Introduction.. xvii

PART I: THE FIRST YEAR

Chapter 1:   Six Reflections on Danny's Diagnosis 3

    Laura *3*

    Brian..*10*

    Jessie *11*

    Danny *11*

    Jack *12*

    Linda *12*

Chapter 2:   Returning Home 14

    The First Trip to the Supermarket..*15*

    The Visiting Nurses Association *16*

    Coping with Mealtimes..*17*

    First Week Food Log...*18*

    Getting Organized..*18*

    Working as a Family Team *20*

    Preparing Friends and Teachers..*22*

Chapter 3:   The First Three Months 25

    The Importance of Educating Yourself *25*

    Finding Additional Care for Danny *29*

Exercise..*32*

A Close Call with My Mother *34*

A Breakthrough with Acupuncture *36*

A Visit to the Emergency Room...*40*

Posttraumatic Stress..*41*

Chapter 4:   The Second Three Months....................44

Getting Away Overnight as a Couple..................................*44*

Trying to Balance the Demands of Work and Home..............*45*

Danny's Honeymoon: Off Insulin!.......................................*48*

Positive Changes in Our Family...*50*

A Typical Day..*51*

Going Camping as a Family *53*

The Challenging Role of Caretaker *54*

Chapter 5:   The Second Six Months 56

Changing Our Diet..*56*

The Roller Coaster Ride: On Insulin Again.........................*59*

Coping with a Fever..*60*

Changing to Another Diabetes Team...................................*62*

An Unexplainable Crisis...*63*

Parties and Halloween..*65*

Working on My Attitude *66*

Danny's Weeklong School Trip..*67*

Meeting Our New Diabetes Team..*69*

Family Meetings...*71*

Helping Siblings Thrive..*72*

PART II: THE SECOND YEAR

Chapter 6:   The First Six Months 75

Our One-Year Anniversary..*75*

Another Family to Lean On *78*

Communicating with Our Doctors......................................*79*

Simplifying Danny's Treatment..80

Hosting a Juvenile Diabetes Research Foundation Coffee...................82

Coping with the Croup 83

Chapter 7:   The Second Sixth Months 86

Danny's Two Weeks at Farm Camp 86

Reflexology...88

Talking about Death with Danny..89

One Week at Family Diabetes Camp 90

The Diabetes Diet War...94

Feelings of Mastery, Finally..95

Our Second Halloween 98

The Be-A-Great-Athlete Approach...99

Losing Faith in Our Second Medical Team......................................102

A Like-Minded Diabetes Team, Finally..103

Chapter 8:   Our Family at Two Years 106

Our Second Christmas 106

A Change in Perspective...107

The Elements of Wonderful Medical Care..108

A Successful Weekend Away 112

Danny's Advice..112

Jessie's Reflections..113

Brian's Philosophy 114

Danny's Final Word on the Subject 116

Chapter 9:   Postscript at Three and One-Half Years (A1c 6.2) .. 117

The Pump..117

Laura: If I Only Knew Then What I Know Now 120

PART III: A SURVIVAL GUIDE FOR PARENTS

Diabetes Preparation 127

Sample Medical Information Sheet..128

Sample Daily Log..129

Getting Support *130*

Family Strategies *131*

Emotional Perspectives *133*

Self-Care *134*

Nutrition *135*

Our Four-day Food Log After Diagnosis *139*

Two-year Food Log *140*

Three-year Food Log *141*

Sources of Information *142*

Glossary of Terms 143

Acknowledgments

This book is complete because of the enthusiasm, love, and support of many. As it made its way from journal to manuscript, Julie and Chris Anderson, Lisa Balis, Annie and Mac Bell, Andrea Bryant, Ra'ufa Clark, Beth Crowe, Dr. Eric Freedland, Shannon Gamble, Drs. Barbara and Ken Holbert, Susan and Pierce Holbert, Melany Kahn, Pat Manson, Lynn Nadeau, Dr. Brian Orr, Christine Ozahowski, Erica Plunkett, Jessica Plunkett, Kaiya Rohrer, Laurie Rosen, Anne Serafin, Amanda Thibert, Ronnie Traynor, and Roberta Xavier put pen to paper and helped my mother and me create this final copy. Special thanks to our editor Clara Schröder, to Mrs. E. S. Kantowicz for her financial support, to Matt Muise for the back cover photo, and to Jane Zeeb and Tom McDonnell for the original cover design and printing advice. Our agent, Charlotte Raymond, had faith and insight from the first draft and her advice sustained and motivated us. Thanks to Nancy Sarles for having a bigger vision than we had...and to Brian Plunkett for making all things possible.

Most importantly, from a mother's point of view, I give my heartfelt gratitude to the people in this book who saw what we needed and stepped in to help.

Foreword
by Dr. Ann Wyttenbach

As a family practitioner with a special interest in diabetes, every day I see the harmful effects of a diet high in refined carbohydrates, simple sugars, and hydrogenated or saturated fats. It is clear to me that as a society we need to change our approach to illness by recognizing the immense impact of nutrition on disease development and control.

The Plunketts' experiences during the first three years following Danny's diagnosis challenge many of the current expectations and treatment plans for children with diabetes. Laura Plunkett trusted her son to understand the connection between good sugar control and how well he felt and functioned, and she secured his cooperation by making him and his sister an integral part of the health care team. Their success demonstrates that children will accept changes in diet and activity levels, if offered with a positive attitude.

In addition, this book confirms that a family can survive and thrive by making their child's illness a family affair, stressing health rather than sickness as motivation. From the author's initial heartbreaking accounts of her challenges to her increasingly positive and affirming achievements, it provides hope to those who doubt that a healthier child and a stronger, healthier family can emerge after a diagnosis of childhood diabetes.

In this story of a family's triumph, I was impressed with Laura Plunkett's refusal to accept elevated blood sugars as normal and expected in childhood diabetes. Questioning conventional medical advice when it didn't work, she had the courage and persistence to proceed by trial and error until she arrived at an optimal plan, both for her son Danny and for her entire family.

Parents will understand and identify with the emotional trauma that accompanies the diagnosis of diabetes in their child. Medical professionals will gain insight into how better to support families. I am not aware of any similarly accessible publication providing the vital information given here. I strongly recommend *The Challenge of Childhood Diabetes* to families and medical practitioners alike.

Ann Wyttenbach, M.D.
Diplomate, American Board of Family Practice

Introduction

When our seven-year-old son, Danny, developed juvenile diabetes, the diagnosis came as a severe shock. One day my husband and I had two active, healthy children; the next, we were faced with the fact that our youngest child had a chronic and life-threatening illness. We were stunned by the enormous impact that diabetes had upon our family. I had an especially difficult time because I felt both very responsible and completely unprepared.

I cried in the supermarket during my first post-diagnosis shopping trip. Breakfast, lunch, and dinner were filled with stress. I wondered how other parents dealt with their confusion and fear, food issues, holidays, and parties. I questioned how others coped with the strain of learning how to make medical decisions, give shots, and do blood tests. I wanted to know how the diagnosed child and his or her siblings felt and how their feelings changed over time. I wanted to be reassured that we would somehow survive the pressure the illness placed on our family and, specifically, on my relationship with my husband.

In those first months, I read every book I could lay my hands on, but I could not find one that described a family's long-term adjustment. I found many how-to books that gave valuable, practical advice, none of which spoke to the ache in my heart or showed how a family could recover its sense of stability, comfort, and hope for the future.

In addition, I looked for information about extending Danny's honeymoon period. After he began getting insulin, his pancreas started producing more insulin on its own. From the moment he needed less insulin, I wanted to extend that stage as long as possible. Although prolonging the honeymoon is an extremely important goal in diabetes research now, at the time no one thought it of any consequence. It seemed to me that helping Danny make as much of his own insulin for as long as he could was far better than injecting a foreign substance, but I could not find any clinicians who had ever tried it.

Since then we have found our own way. Through trial and error, our family made sense of overwhelming and often conflicting advice about nutrition. We developed a kid-friendly whole-foods diet that keeps Danny's blood sugar levels from spiking or dropping too quickly and keeps all of us healthy, energized, and at an optimum weight. We found many ways to enjoy exercising with Danny, which helps keep his numbers low. We also incorporated complementary care such as acupuncture and acupressure, as a way to support Danny's endocrine system, with very beneficial results. We kept searching until we found a medical team that fit our family and, ultimately, helped us make the transition from injections to the insulin pump.

Making decisions based on what fit our family has paid off. Danny's honeymoon lasted almost two years, and his insulin needs continue to be lower than normal for his age and weight. While the average child with juvenile diabetes has a Hemoglobin A1c number (representing the average of blood sugar levels of the previous three months) of 8.5, and one-third of American children are above 9.5, in the past nine months, Danny's numbers have been 6.2 and 6.3. This is important because the American Diabetes Association and the American Academy of Endocrinologists recommend staying under 7.0 and 6.5, respectively, to avoid or minimize long-term complications.

Danny is now stronger physically, at an ideal weight, more consistently rested, healthier, more resistant to colds and flu (this winter none of us were sick at all), and more vibrantly alive than he has ever been, but I still wish I'd been able to find diabetes books that talked about creating overall health. I was looking for support in treating the whole child, not just the disease. A challenge like diabetes should invite you to try to improve your child's life in *every* way. During the last two years, as I improvised ways to help him, I often struggled with the doubting voice in my head because I did not have any role models.

Three years ago, as we struggled with uncontrollable blood sugar levels, lack of sleep, and the sudden onslaught of so many new demands, everyone seemed to have a horror story about seizures, comas, or the long-term complications associated with diabetes. I had many fears for Danny and for our ten-year-old daughter, Jessie. I was afraid that the focus we put on Danny would make Jessie feel neglected or drive her away. Would this disease tear our family apart?

In hindsight, I can see that by "circling the wagons," by letting diabetes take center stage in the beginning, our family slowly and deliberately developed a new way of being. By curtailing our outside interests and focusing so much attention on mastering Danny's care, meeting Jessie's needs, and strengthening our marriage, we created a safe "home base" where we slowly developed a new definition of a "normal" life.

At this point, Danny takes part in sports, goes on sleepovers, and is happy and successful at school. Despite my worst fears, he has never gone into a coma or awakened throwing up. He doesn't seem sorry for himself, nor is he self-destructive, passive-aggressive, teased, or excluded from activities by other children. Although initially an incredibly picky eater whose main diet consisted of pasta, white bread, juice, and desserts, he now enjoys a wider range of the healthy foods that make up our relatively low-carbohydrate diet. Whatever his teen years bring, we are grateful for today's smooth sailing.

We are also aware that diabetes comes with its own gifts though I could never have imagined myself saying that when Danny was first diagnosed. Jessie, at age fourteen, has become Danny's best babysitter. Because of our new diet and a greater emphasis on exercise, she is healthier and thinner than she was before. Although she has had to mature quickly, learning to be a team player has held her in good stead at home and at school. She does not seem to have suffered from the event that divided our life into before and after. My husband and I have learned to rely upon each other in ways we had never done before, and we are grateful for good times with an intensity we would never have felt if we weren't facing this challenge together.

Obviously, at the beginning, I knew none of this. Overwhelmed and anxious all the time, I needed an outlet for my emotions, a way to reflect upon my experiences and the tremendous amount of information I was absorbing. Luckily, my parents live around the corner, and at random times I found myself sharing what was happening with my mother, who is a writer. Over the next two years, I described the rewarding and heartbreaking moments of Danny's illness, without self-consciousness or censorship. My mother listened and typed while I thought things through aloud. It took two years before our family reached a point where I felt we had constructed a way of life that felt not only manageable but also hopeful and happy.

At that point, we were surprised to find we had 250 pages describing our journey from a family mired in shock and apprehension to our current state—stable, confident, and conscious of our many blessings. I became convinced that others just entering this frightening world could benefit from our story. I wanted to share what we had finally distilled from our experience, to describe our accomplishments and our blunders so that the learning curve for others would be easier than the one we faced. In an effort to include more perspectives, my mother,

Linda, added her own entries and interviewed my husband, Brian, my son, Danny, my daughter, Jessie, and my father, Jack.

This book offers no easy answers. Instead, it reveals the slow maturing of a family struggling to maintain a balance between caring and overprotection, between self-discipline and self-indulgence, and between being loving parents and loving partners. We believe that validation—knowing that another family has successfully coped with impersonal doctors and sudden fevers, with Halloween and birthday parties, with sibling jealousy and the sudden loss of every carefree moment—makes the process of healing easier.

The story of our life with Danny is not meant to be a definition of the "right way" to achieve this. All we hope to do is show you our way and encourage you to find yours. Although we have created a summary of all the lessons we learned in the section titled "A Survival Guide for Parents," we have found, over time, that in the moments when we paused and looked closely at what was happening, when we listened to what *we* thought and what *we* wanted, we found important answers and got the best results.

When you become pregnant, people can tell you what it is like to give birth, but no one can prepare you. Your old life dissolves, and you are forced by love and circumstance to step up to the plate and be a parent. In the same way, when your child gets diabetes, no matter how much you read about it, you will be taken aback by the reality. Your old life dissolves, and this time, as the parent of a child with diabetes, routines and family patterns need to be formed all over again. Without having a choice, you become someone who thinks about ketones and blood sugar levels, someone who lives in a constant state of vigilance, and someone who bears the daily responsibility for a child's life or death.

Parents of children with diabetes long to take this new unsettled life and right themselves again. We all want to reach that place where a child's diabetes is no longer such a huge blow to our equilibrium. We want to be comfortable with a new definition of normal. Though it is hard to imagine incorporating diabetes into your lifestyle so deeply that it becomes an integral part of who you are as a family, that is what happens over time.

It is important, however, not to underestimate how stressful the adjustment can be. I had countless advantages: an involved husband, a loving extended family, comprehensive health insurance, and enough money to take a prolonged leave of absence from work after Danny was diagnosed. Yet, I still had feelings I hope I never feel again.

A recent study on posttraumatic stress disorder (PTSD) in parents of children with newly diagnosed Type 1 diabetes found that 24 percent of the mothers and 22 percent of the fathers met full diagnostic criteria for posttraumatic stress disorder. In addition, in the first year after diagnosis, mothers of newly diagnosed children become clinically depressed two to three times more often than other mothers.

Unfortunately, few people realize how much parents need support. One of the most isolating aspects of having a child with diabetes is that friends and relatives often fail to comprehend the enormous demands diabetes makes upon a family and assume that everything has returned to normal within two or three months. Since children with diabetes do not look ill, it is easy for others to forget the very thing that consumes a parent's life. When friends read early copies of my manuscript, they immediately responded with greater sympathy and understanding. I no longer felt excluded from the community of the healthy by their incomprehension. Perhaps by sharing this book and your own experiences with others, you will be able to bridge the gap between your life and theirs.

Many of your reactions will not be the same as mine, but if you feel as if you will never reach solid ground, please know that you are not alone. You will regain your sense of balance as time passes. Although some families may recover sooner than we did, even slow learners discover unknown strengths.

In any moment when accepting this illness seems beyond your reach, you can also take a vacation from the "facts" and simply watch your child. Whether he is reading a book or she is tying her shoes, our children are extraordinary, whole, and alive. We have them now, and in every moment when the details and distractions can be set aside, it is enough.

PART I

▼

The First Year

CHAPTER 1

▼

Six Reflections on Danny's Diagnosis

Laura

I stood in a strange living room with the phone to my ear, hearing our family doctor tell me that my healthy, active son might be seriously ill.

"Listen, I can't bear this," I felt like saying. "You have to take it back. Our family just can't handle it right now." Yet here it was, no matter what we did, another day, another crisis.

It was the first Saturday in January 2002. My husband Brian and I had escaped to a rental home in Southern Maine with our ten year-old daughter, Jessie, and our seven-year-old son, Danny, to recover from the crippling tensions of the fall, but life had its own agenda.

Our luck wasn't changing.

It had all started in August, five months earlier, when a car had struck Danny. On the third day of our vacation at the beach, he was standing by the side of the road next to his dad. Without warning, and without any sense of why he had done it, he stepped backward in front of a white station wagon traveling at thirty miles an hour. I was below the road on the bank of an inlet, looking for crabs with Jessie. There was a terrible squeal of brakes, and I looked up to see Danny rolling down the road in his red-and-yellow bathing shorts, arms and legs flailing. I scrambled up the rocky bank to the sound of my own screaming, scraping my hands and knees without feeling a thing. Witnesses later told me that he had been

- 3 -

thrown onto the hood and into the air, then landed on his head on the pavement before rolling twenty feet. By the time I got to him, he was covered in blood.

When the emergency crew arrived, they pushed back the crowd and strapped Danny to a board. They put him quickly into the back of the ambulance and allowed me to ride with him. I held his hand and concentrated on my breathing while Brian and Jessie followed in our car, getting lost on the way. Just after the EMT called the local hospital and told the emergency room that Danny was a Code 3—the worst—Danny moved his oxygen mask from his face, looked up at me, and whispered, "Don't worry, Mommy. I'm fine."

For several hours, we didn't know the extent of Danny's injuries. Jessie, Brian, and I stood by his hospital litter while he remained strapped to the board for a half-day of tests, including a CT scan and full-body x-rays. He was bloody and bruised but fully conscious and calm. We matched his mood as best we could, and Jessie promised him presents to make up for all his pain and suffering. In the end, we were told he had only a slight concussion and road burn. Danny might have been killed, but except for some serious bruises, he seemed to have escaped with little harm.

Anyone who has come that close to losing a child knows that it takes a long time to feel normal again. The rest of our vacation was a blur of bandages and ointments, doctor's visits, and persistent anxiety. Brian and I clung to each other at night, stunned by the sheer immensity of how close we'd just come to having our hearts blown apart. Jessie was tearful and clingy. She developed an earache, and her eardrum burst. All of a sudden, life felt like a tightrope, and all four of us worried that someone was going to topple off. Even weeks later, we were holding the kids' hands in parking lots and warning them to be careful as we were crossing the street.

On a Saturday in October, by the time my fears were starting to ease, Danny fell off his skateboard while at a friend's house and loosened his front, permanent teeth. My neighbor brought him to the door, bloody and shaken, and Brian and I rushed him to our dentist, Dr. Corrine Barone. While Dr. Barone dug the gravel out of his lip and built braces to reset his teeth, I huddled in a corner of the room. Calm until he was in her care, I was now shaking with adrenaline and woozy with nausea. I kept telling myself that this wasn't life-and-death, that I'd come a long way from the scene of the car accident, but I couldn't relax. Brian handled the payment, made the follow-up appointments, and we headed home. That night, after dreaming that Danny was slipping out of my grasp and falling, I woke up with my heart pounding.

In November and December, both kids had several colds and the flu. Jessie alone got strep throat, stomach flu, and pneumonia. There were too many trips to the doctor's office and not enough days in school. After the holidays and school vacation week, we were all more depleted than we'd ever been. If we survived the holiday rush, we vowed we'd take a long weekend away and do absolutely nothing.

We arrived at our rented house late on the Friday after New Year's Eve. All of our hard times were behind us, we hoped. We dragged our bags as far as the doorway of each bedroom, brushed our teeth, and murmured good night. Saturday morning, we woke late and explored, sleepily moving from room to room in our pajamas. The kids eagerly searched through the basket of children's books and the closet brimming with games and puzzles.

Brian and I made a pot of coffee and admired the snow-covered hill out the window. Sitting in the kitchen, we talked about everything that came to mind: his work as a lawyer and what he wanted from his career; my job as a part-time counselor and how I could better juggle the roles of mother, therapist, and wife; the weather; our children's school; a friend's divorce. Even after nineteen years of loving each other, we sometimes felt lonely, the demands of family having come between us until we were reduced to catching up with each other in quick phone conversations and late-night talks. By lunchtime, however, the familiar comfort and warmth between us that always came from unhurried conversation was back.

As we fixed a spaghetti lunch, the kids spotted the deep snow on the hill across the street. They grabbed two sleds from a closet in the hall and rushed out the door. As I watched from the kitchen window, Jessie climbed the hill, stopping to grab her brother's mittened hand. Danny shook her off and charged up the hill past her, eager to beat his older sister to the top. I watched her run after him, relieved, after a long run of illnesses, to have two healthy children.

To my surprise, the phone rang. Who would be calling us here? Reluctantly, I took the call. It was our family doctor, Dr. Len Horowitz, who immediately apologized for interrupting our vacation with the results of Danny's blood and urine tests. Right before Christmas, Danny had started wetting his bed at night. He hadn't done that since he was three, but Brian and I took it in stride, assuming he had a simple urinary tract infection. I had brought him in for routine tests at a local hospital just before our family left for Maine. I thanked our doctor for tracking us down, assuming he would prescribe some antibiotics.

After a pause, he said, "Danny's blood sugar levels are high. Unfortunately, you need to come home."

It was my turn to hesitate. "Blood sugar?" I had no idea what that meant.

Dr. Horowitz said, "High blood sugar levels could indicate several things, some of them serious, and you need to be close to home until we figure out what the results mean."

Brian was watching me with his coffee cup poised halfway to his mouth. I shook my head and waved off his concern. "There must be some mistake. Lab tests can be wrong."

Dr. Horowitz asked me about Danny's symptoms. "Does he seem lethargic? Listless? Is he overly thirsty or urinating frequently? Is there anything unusual about his behavior?"

I looked out the window again with a restored sense of calm. "He's currently charging up a hill with his sister, dragging a sled. He's always hungry and thirsty. That's the story of his life. And we haven't noticed anything unusual except the bed-wetting, which he didn't do last night."

You have to understand. Life was about to get immeasurably easier. Brian and I had just discussed ways we could simplify our schedules. I was going to quit my position as the head of the site-search committee for the kids' school. Brian was going to limit his marketing efforts at work to lunches and seminars, so he'd only be out at night for his martial arts class. We'd decided to limit each child to only one activity outside of school commitments. With everyone healthy, we were off to a promising start.

"I am sure there was a mistake in the lab tests," I now said to the doctor. "How about if we promise to bring him for tests before school Monday morning?"

Dr. Horowitz paused briefly, and then relented. "As long as you call me the minute you notice a change in Danny's behavior. I'll see you in two days."

On the morning of January 7, Danny and I arrived at our local hospital for his second blood and urine analysis. After the test, I dropped him off at school. He'd wet the bed again the night before, but he seemed fine, and neither of us was worried. At eleven o'clock, however, Dr. Horowitz called me at home.

"Laura," he said, a grave tone in his voice, "I'm sorry to tell you that Danny has diabetes."

It's hard to believe now, but I laughed. Even though Dr. Horowitz had been our doctor for seven years and I trusted him implicitly, I was sure he was overreacting. Danny couldn't be seriously ill. Moreover, he couldn't have diabetes. All I knew about diabetes was that this was a disease where parents had to give their kids shots. I could never do that. There had to be some mistake.

I decided I must not be communicating clearly enough.

"He can't have diabetes," I said, "because he is completely healthy."

Dr. Horowitz recognized denial when he saw it. "Where is Danny now?" he asked.

"At school," I replied.

Now he was authoritative. "Pack a bag full of his clothes and a stuffed animal. Go get him at school and bring him to the hospital. He needs immediate care."

I felt my first wave of panic. I didn't want to believe that my family was in trouble. I made a last attempt to keep things normal. "Danny was fine when I left him this morning. Can't we wait 'til the end of the school day?"

"No."

It was too much to bear. The car. The skateboard. Now, for the third time in six months, I couldn't protect my son.

As I dialed the number for Danny's school, I started to cry uncontrollably. I've always thought of myself as someone who holds it together under stress, and yet I couldn't complete the call without help. I walked straight to my mother's house two blocks away and burst in on her. Blessedly, she was home, and as I climbed the stairs and heard her voice, I became hysterical.

Despite the tears, I knew I had to get Danny medical help as soon as possible. With my mom standing next to me, I called the school. The secretary went into Danny's classroom and returned to tell me that he had just finished telling his teacher, "I feel as if I could sleep for a thousand weeks." Now I was scared. I hadn't packed. I hadn't called Brian. I didn't know what to do with Jessie.

I called my father Jack, a child psychiatrist, whose office is nearby. Luckily, he's calm in emergencies. I tearfully told him the bare bones of the story, and he offered to cancel his patients and pick up my children at school. He organized me: I was to go home, pack Danny's clothes, and wait for him so we could all drive to the hospital together.

I went home and tried to pack. I was so distraught that after I'd chosen a pair of Danny's pajamas, I came to a standstill, unable to decide which stuffed animal to choose. I reached for the phone and called my friend and neighbor, Ronnie. She was at my house in two minutes and talked me through a checklist to make sure I took everything Danny might need. Soon after, my mother, my father, and my kids arrived at our house, and we drove into the hospital where Brian met us in the emergency room.

I was in a state of shock. I couldn't see how Danny could possibly go from a healthy, energetic child to a boy with a chronic illness overnight. We all chatted and reassured one another, while Danny lay on an examining table in a cubicle and waited for the doctors and nurses. The initial tests and examinations took all afternoon. I still didn't know what juvenile diabetes was, but I didn't want to ask questions in front of the kids.

We were told there were no beds available; we'd have to wait until another patient left the hospital. Everything seemed to be moving in slow motion with an unreal quality to it, especially since I was pretending to be calm and unconcerned so that Danny wouldn't be scared. By dinnertime, he was settled in a double room with a roommate, a boy with hemophilia.

As soon as Danny was given a room, we began a three-day educational program while the hospital staff tried to stabilize Danny's blood sugars. We were assigned a nutritionist, a therapist, a nurse diabetes educator, and several admitting physicians, and told we would meet with all of these people during our stay. The first part of our education started that night, out of Danny's hearing, when all of a sudden I was confronted with the enormity and complexity of this disease. The doctors said that Danny would need three to six injections each day, five to eight blood glucose tests, and seven carefully calculated meals and snacks. Then they also told us that as soon as he started on insulin, he would be at risk of lapsing into a seizure or a coma.

My mind went dark, and unbearable thoughts blotted out every word after that. *If I made a mistake in judgment, my son could die.* All I could focus on was that the insulin needed to keep him alive could also kill him. I found myself sobbing and unable to stop in front of people I had never met before. I'm a fairly private person, but there was no secluded place to get myself together except the bathroom.

In this intense state of grief and disorientation, my husband and I began a series of educational training sessions on the fundamentals of diabetes. Jessie calmly joined us in the meetings, and armed with a pencil and paper, asked many of the questions I was too numb to ask. There were handouts on diet planning, different types of insulin, carbohydrate counting, giving injections, blood sugar monitoring, how to recognize and treat seizures and comas, the role of exercise, and the long-term consequences of the disease. Fear, like static, disturbed my ability to listen. I felt as if I would never master all this information. Danny would come home, and I wouldn't know what to do.

That first night my parents left, and Brian took Jessie home. I stayed in the hospital and lay on a vinyl chair that doubled as a bed, but I barely slept. The alarms on the machines attached to Danny's roommate went off every forty-five minutes. By morning, I was bleary-eyed, still in shock and emotionally and physically exhausted.

At six thirty, a nurse came in with a cheerful hello and asked if I was ready to give Danny his first insulin shot of the day. Speechless, I shook my head no and backed away, rebelling at the thought that on my first try I would be using my child as a guinea pig. Danny was incredibly brave, but as I watched the nurse give the shot for me, I'm embarrassed to say I was the one who cried.

When my father arrived that evening, he asked the nurse for saline and syringes and cheerfully let all of us, including my mom and my daughter, practice giving him shots in the arm. Even Danny got a chance to inject his willing grandfather with saline water. None of us had much trouble giving a shot to my dad who smiled throughout and kept saying, "Aw, that didn't hurt."

That first full day was also difficult because food service was overwhelmed and frequently sent up the wrong food or left us waiting for Danny's tray at mealtimes. We had been told that the timing and content of Danny's meals were vitally important, so Brian and I rushed around frantically trying to get hold of the proper food seven times a day. The nurses let Danny pick from the menu, and he chose grilled cheese, macaroni and cheese, chicken nuggets, sugar-free Jell-O, and diet soda. Our family avoided processed and fried foods. I was vaguely aware that he was eating worse food here than he did at home.

On the second day, the sterile room, the hospital food, and the harried pace began to wear on us. Danny seemed numb to everything. The kid who watched television or played computer games only on weekends now watched television or was engrossed in the hospital's portable PlayStation every waking moment. He barely talked to us. He didn't ask questions, and his only complaint was that he hated the needles, though he passively submitted when the nurses came in to give him shots. We couldn't seem to reach him. The child whose face was usually alive with a twinkle of mischief was missing in action.

People came in and out of his room throughout the day: nurses, aides, doctors, residents, nutritionists, cleaners, food servers, and family visitors. The constant interruptions didn't leave us time to be together as a family. I was having trouble keeping track of who all these people were; I couldn't remember faces. Most taxing was trying not to cry. I didn't want the kids to panic, and I didn't want to call attention to myself. That night I went home with Jessie to try to get a good night's sleep, leaving Brian to keep watch. At ten that evening, a baby with burns became Danny's new roommate and cried all night long. Brian, stretched out on the vinyl chair, didn't sleep at all.

On the morning of the third day, we met Dr. C who said he'd be our endocrinologist outside the hospital. He urged us to stay another night so we could learn more about the disease. He said that the staff was concerned about me because I was so tearful and suggested I use that time to see the therapist. We told him that we wanted to go home. The sleepless nights, our lack of control, and the lack of privacy to talk things over seemed intolerable. We felt that we'd rather deal with our own fears and try to explain things to the kids in our own home. Brian and I were both so adamant that we convinced Dr. C to discharge us. We promised we'd immediately set up a meeting with the local Visiting Nurses Association.

I took one month of prescriptions down to the pharmacy in the hospital lobby. The co-pay for the first month was $260. I left with a bag full of pharmaceuticals: syringes, alcohol wipes, lancets, insulin, glucose monitors, and test strips, along with doubts about my ability to use any of them. I felt weak and scared, holding on to my veneer of calm as tightly as I was gripping the pharmacy bag. It was taking everything I had just to put one foot in front of another, but Brian, who'd been like a rock throughout the whole experience, was convinced we could do it.

We packed up and went home.

Brian

A week later, Brian and I finally had some time alone, and we talked about how he'd felt that first day.

"After you called and told me that the doctor was insisting that you take Danny directly to the hospital, I left work immediately so I could take part in the check-in process. On the way over I was thinking, 'This is bad,' but very vaguely because I didn't know much about diabetes. Like most people, I didn't realize the effort involved. I figured Danny might have to have a shot now and then and wouldn't be able to eat sugar."

The admission process seemed fine to him even though there was a lot of waiting around until they finally admitted us. "Those first few days went by in a whirlwind, with the hospital trying to cram everything into us that we needed to know before we could bring Danny home. I didn't feel shaken until I got home with Jessie that first night, after leaving you two at the hospital. I stayed up that night reading the booklet they gave us and tried to absorb all the bad things that could happen. I couldn't believe how suddenly our life had changed."

By the end of that week, Brian was feeling less scared and less despondent. "I had no choice. Despite the chaos of the hospital stay, I was able to focus and I felt that they'd given us the information we needed. I actually felt pretty confident that we could manage Danny's diabetes if we just took things one day at a time. You always look ahead to see what the impact is going to be, and you could see this was going to be huge. You were so overwhelmed that it felt really important that I remain calm.

"I remember thinking, 'Why us?' I ended up concluding that God chose us because God knows that we can do this. We each have our own path in life, and dealing with diabetes is Danny's path, and dealing with Danny having diabetes is our path, for whatever reason."

Jessie

Around the same time, I asked Jessie what that day was like for her.

"When Grandpa knocked on the door of my fifth-grade classroom in the middle of class, my Spanish teacher opened the door and said, 'Jessie, come here.'

"I was puzzled. Who would want me in the middle of Spanish? When I saw it was Poppop, I was even more confused. He told me we needed to take Danny to the hospital. I didn't even know Danny was sick.

"I didn't know why I had to come if Danny was the one who was sick, but in the car you said it was because no one would be home to meet me after school. None of us talked much during the drive, but Poppop did tell me that Danny might have diabetic problems. I knew what diabetes was because when I was nine, a girl at my day camp had it. Danny complained about having to get a blood test all the way to the hospital.

"Once we got there, we met Daddy in the lobby and then sat in the waiting room for about fifteen minutes before we went into a little cubicle and a doctor looked at Danny. Then we all waited for what seemed like hours. I got bored so Nana took me to a bookstore, and I got a Calvin and Hobbes comic book for Danny. When we got back to the hospital, he was upstairs.

"We all stayed in his room for a while. When you decided to stay in the hospital with Danny, I went home with Dad. It was weird going home and leaving you there. The next morning Dad and I drove back to the hospital. Danny was happy playing video games. I went downstairs to the drugstore with you. You called Ronnie and I stood in the lobby listening to your conversation. You were crying. That was when I realized this wasn't going to be just an overnight thing.

"I'm glad you explained everything to me after that, and let me skip school again to come back to the hospital for diabetes classes the next day. Learning all about how to give shots and how to test Danny's blood sugar was definitely more fun than school."

Danny

At dinner one night, Danny told a friend what happened.

"I was wetting my bed and I was really thirsty a lot, so I had a blood test and the results came back. My grandpa came and knocked on my door at school and took me home. My mom told me I had diabetes, so we packed me up and went to the hospital. I had never heard of diabetes before. I could barely even say the name. When we got there, we did all this stuff and then they took me to my room. I wasn't really scared, but every time I got a shot it really killed." He paused for effect. "Grandpa said we could practice giving shots on him. We took the needle and drew up a saline solution and we gave him shots to practice. I liked that. After a while, it didn't hurt so much when I had to get a shot.

"I liked playing with all the games at the hospital. They had this room at the end of the hall, which was filled with games and stuff, and my parents let me watch television all the time. It was pretty fun."

Jack

My father described going into robot mode, something he learned in medical school and has perfected in years of practice. He didn't think about how he felt. He focused instead on all the details of getting his grandchildren into town without scaring Danny. He decided to stop at a 7-11 for a treat to give the ride the feeling of an "adventure."

When he got to the hospital, he only let a little of the medical reality sink in. His attention as a doctor was directed at how well the hospital staff was handling things. Actually, he was surprised at how much he didn't know about diet and the various tests Danny would have to go through. A lot had changed in the forty years since he went to medical school.

"I felt like Danny and I were part of a rejectionist front. Neither one of us was willing to think of this as a big deal, even though we both knew it was. He was concentrating on his PlayStation, and I was focusing on logistics. My proudest accomplishment is that by the end of that day I got everyone, including Danny, comfortable giving shots, a hurdle which takes some families months."

Linda

My mother was sitting in front of her computer, updating her phone list, when I burst into the room. I don't think I've cried in my mother's presence since I was a teenager, but the minute I tried to speak I was wracked with such explosive sobs that she couldn't understand the sounds coming out of my mouth. She just stood up, put her arms around me, and held on.

She finally made out the words, "Danny" and "diabetes." She almost laughed. Since Danny didn't eat junk food, was fairly thin, and had no family risk factors, she was sure this whole thing was a mistake. Finally, I got the whole story out. When she asked, "Are you sure?" it set off another round of inconsolable crying so she focused on just being there and saying little, feeling that the last thing she should do was to add her own wild feelings to the tempest.

As we were all waiting in the hospital lobby, she realized that she could distract Jessie, so the two of them headed to a nearby bookstore to look for something funny for Danny to read. She told me how surreal it felt to be looking at books as if she and Jessie were ordinary people having an ordinary day while just down the street our own personal nightmare seemed to be unfolding.

"My mother got diabetes in her seventies," she told me. "It didn't seem like a big deal. She was overweight and simply went on eating candy, but this was different. Juvenile diabetes is treatable, but it's also incurable, chronic, and life-threatening. It felt unbearable to think that this time the patient was a seven-year-old boy who couldn't fully understand what had happened, never mind cope with it."

As she sat in on all the conferences, she learned that the treatment of juvenile diabetes was anything but cut-and-dried. She realized that keeping Danny healthy would require a high level of mathematical and problem-solving skills, constant vigilance for signs of high or low blood sugar levels, excellent management skills, and steadfast attention to whether he was complying with dietary restrictions. She felt like she needed a college course to master it all. Having recently been diagnosed with Adult Attention Deficit Disorder, she felt particularly ill-suited to handle his care.

Yet that second night in the hospital, as we all jabbed my dad, she managed to overcome a lifetime fear of needles. "When Danny got on his knees on the bed and stuck Jack with enormous pleasure," she said, "for the first time he seemed to me like the boy I'd known, not a zombie in a hospital bed mesmerized by television and electronic games. On the third day, when you and Brian gave Danny his shots, and he stopped tensing up and clenching his teeth, for the first time I thought, *this might be doable.*"

CHAPTER 2

▼

Returning Home

During our hospital stay, we mastered the following fundamentals about juvenile diabetes: Insulin is made in our bodies by islet or beta cells, which reside in the pancreas. When we eat carbohydrates and/or protein, the body turns some of this food into sugar in the bloodstream. The pancreas secretes insulin to allow the excess sugar to move out of the blood and into the cells of the body. When we're not eating, our islet cells don't produce a lot of insulin.

Current theory says that in a growing percentage of children an unknown virus or event triggers a genetic predisposition to diabetes. The autoimmune system then starts attacking the body's insulin-producing cells. Over a series of months or years, the number of islet cells decreases until a child begins to have too much sugar in his or her blood. The child enters a state called ketoacidosis and exhibits overt symptoms such as extreme thirst, frequent urination, fatigue, and weight loss. If the diabetes goes undetected, the child becomes extremely ill and ultimately collapses into a coma. To remedy the problem of too much sugar in the blood, children get manufactured insulin through injections or from a pump worn at the waist.

In order for Brian and me to know how much insulin to give Danny at any given moment, we had to prick his skin and test his current blood sugar level with a meter, count the amount of carbohydrates about to be eaten, consider the amount of recent or expected exercise, and then select a dose. Insulin and exercise both reduce blood sugar levels. Stress, illness, hormonal changes, food, and certain medications increase it. When we first learned this, we had the sense that we'd have some control over what Danny's numbers would be, but we came to realize that we couldn't predict his numbers, even if his life depended on it. And it did.

We arrived home on a Wednesday night hoping to keep Danny's numbers between the doctors' recommended goal range of 80 to 180. At eight o'clock, he was 360. In the following forty-eight hours, we tested Danny's blood sugars every four hours and only saw the "right numbers" three times.

The First Trip to the Supermarket

Once we were home, we all seemed to be running on adrenaline. Danny got three shots per day, which took us an interminable amount of time to calculate, draw up, and inject. He ate seven times a day, and Brian and I spent hours looking up how many carbohydrates were in each ingredient or item. We doled out his food with cup measures as instructed by the nutritionist. We started testing his blood sugars every two hours. I was nervous all the time.

My first outing was to the supermarket, and I entered the store feeling relieved to be out of the house for a while. The fruit and vegetable aisle was easy, and I stocked up on all the regulars: lettuce, cucumbers, carrots, apples, bananas, and a few pears. Dairy was uneventful. Then I turned down the cookie and cracker aisle. Carbohydrates galore and Danny could only have fifteen to thirty at each snack. I found the graham crackers and looked at the nutritional label: three halves for fifteen carbohydrates. Add a glass of milk and that would be it. Even though I was determined to be upbeat and make this a learning adventure, I couldn't help thinking, *that's not enough food for a growing boy.*

I shook my head and moved to the Pepperidge Farm goldfish, a family staple. Fifteen carbohydrates would allow Danny forty-five crackers, about three or four handfuls. I tried to picture him counting the fish. I couldn't imagine it. *No one really does that, do they?* He could have six Ritz crackers, six to twelve tortilla chips, eight animal crackers. Obviously, no one knew my son and his appetite. *How can I offer him six saltines with a straight face?*

I started to panic.

A woman came toward me, chatting with the toddler in her cart. She absent-mindedly reached for a bag of chips, a few boxes of cookies, and some crackers. She laughed at something her child said and excused herself as she moved past me. I was suddenly so saddened that I had to get away. I moved to another aisle where I checked out the ketchup: four carbohydrates per tablespoon. Danny drowns his hot dogs in ketchup. Peanut butter was three carbohydrates per table-spoon, and jelly was nine. I had just learned that a slice of bread was approximately fifteen. That made one of Danny's standard peanut butter and jelly sandwiches fifty carbohydrates, almost all of his allowance for lunch.

Now I was starting to cry in the supermarket, and I never cry in public. I pretended to look at the tomato sauce. When I could focus again, I realized that tomato sauce has nine carbohydrates for a half-cup. Danny could no longer just slosh it on and enjoy. It was definitely time to go. I ended up throwing a bag of popcorn (fifteen carbs for three cups) and some almonds (five carbs for a ¼ cup) in the cart and headed for the checkout counter.

What I needed at that moment was another mother who'd been through this, who could have calmly told me what I know now: that my son would learn to eat a wider range of foods; that he wouldn't starve to death or develop eating disorders; and that we were on the road, rough as it was, to something manageable. Without anyone to turn to, I cried all the way home.

I sat in the driveway until I got myself together. I told myself that somehow other parents manage, though I didn't know any. I assumed that somehow we'd figure it out. Deep inside, however, I felt the elemental pain of knowing that our way of being a family was shattered forever. Then I took a deep breath and brought my single bag of groceries inside.

The Visiting Nurses Association

The visiting nurses were a godsend. As I entered the house, our primary nurse, Robert, was explaining to Brian that he had a daughter with juvenile diabetes himself. He gave us a sunny picture of how well children could live with this disease. He told us that he was closer to his daughter because of her diabetes and that you actually do reach a point when it's all second nature. Autopilot sounded great to me. Robert was funny and extremely knowledgeable, and he talked to Danny directly. He visited us twice a week for a month.

We also had a very helpful and caring VNA nutritionist named Mary. She spent hours with us over a period of weeks, setting us up with a food plan based on Danny's pre-diabetes tastes and needs, then adjusting it as we watched him gain weight. She fit his favorites—bagels, pasta, and juice—into his meal plan. She also described research into promising technologies that would make diabetes easier to deal with in the future, so her visits were reassuring.

Having the VNA nurses helped us manage many "firsts." At one point Mary took a brochure from her bag and slid it across the table to me. It was a catalogue with medical alert bracelets. I looked up and our eyes locked. All right, now I had a child who needed everyone to know he needed help.

"Hey, Danny," I said brightly. "Come choose a medical alert bracelet. They let people know you're on insulin in case there's an emergency."

The bands came in tie-dye, leopard, paisley, leather, and solid colors. He leaned over the photos. "Can I have any one I want?"

I nodded, worried that this would make him feel different from the other kids.

He picked a brown leather strap, saying, "This one's cool. Thanks!" and I realized it was my hang-up.

His teacher later told me that Danny showed his class the medallion with "Insulin Dependent Diabetes" in small print and several of the boys wanted one.

Coping with Mealtimes

Even though Danny quickly adjusted to shots and blood tests, mealtimes were never easy. He was a notoriously stubborn and uncooperative eater who only liked very specific foods, like Annie's macaroni and cheese and Skippy peanut butter. In the past we'd put a meal in front of him, and if he didn't like it after he'd tasted it, he could make himself a sandwich. Now he had to eat every bite at every meal to prevent the insulin we'd given him from bringing his blood sugar below safe levels.

At the initial diagnosis, the hospital nutritionist had put Danny on a diet of 335-350 carbohydrates a day because his weight had fallen to eighty-three pounds on his four-foot, six-inch frame, a loss of eight pounds. This meant he started the day with four or five pancakes and imitation sugar-free syrup, had several grilled cheese sandwiches and carrot sticks for lunch, and meat and potatoes or macaroni and cheese for dinner. Not to mention four snacks. Even though it was obviously too much food, Brian and I deferred to the expertise of the medical team and convinced our reluctant child to eat after he was full.

I kept a log during the first four days we were home, when we seemed to be constantly on the phone with doctors about Danny's high numbers, stomachaches, headaches, fatigue, facial tics, and aches and pains in his arms and legs.

Our First Night Home—Wednesday, January 9, 2002:

8:00 Danny has stomachache, headache, very hyper, very tired, facial tics, blood sugar (BS) 360
Called doctor on call—he said add 2.5 Humalog, 4.5 NPH (insulin)
9:40 BS 314, complaining of aches and pains in legs and arms
9:50 asleep
10:37 BS 315, called doctor on call, Danny wet bed

First Week Food Log

*c = carbohydrate **BS = blood sugar level

Day total c=335-350	Thursday 1-10	Friday 1-11	Saturday 1-12	Sunday 1-13
Breakfast 75c	large bagel with butter 1 c. protein shake **called doctor on call (doc) BS 150 Dan—shaky, achy, not hungry**	large bagel w butter 1 c. protein shake **BS 220**	5 pancakes sugar-free syrup **BS 201**	4 pancakes sugar-free syrup milk
AM Snack 30c	1/2 5" cantaloupe 1 cup milk	popcorn	banana cantaloupe	snack mix
Lunch 60c	German pancake roasted almonds applesauce milk **called doc BS 338**	2 slices pizza cookie **BS 178**	1 & 1/2 grilled cheese milk red pepper **called doc BS 379**	1 & 1/2 grilled cheese milk red pepper/carrots
2:30 Snack 20c	pineapple sugar-free Jell-O water	Apple	Apple	bag of Doritos
4:00 Snack 40c	milk roasted almonds **BS 350**	1/2 c. ice cream 1 c. milk **Dan—hungry, achy, cold, tired**	3/4 c. pretzel mix	2 oz. Cornbread protein shake
Dinner 80c	1 chicken breast 1 & 1/2 c. noodles with butter **called doc**	6 pieces sushi ribs **called doc BS 259**	German pancake snack mix carrots cucumber milk	2 c. noodles with butter parmesan cheese **called doc**
PM Snack 30-45c depending on BS**	popcorn 8 pretzels milk **called doc BS 145 Dan—achy, hungry**	popcorn milk **BS 179**	bread & butter milk **called doc**	cantaloupe milk

When Danny started getting pudgy, I asked our visiting nutritionist to come and talk to him. She asked him what he liked to eat and convinced him to add a few vegetables to his long list of high-carbohydrate foods. We ended up with a new meal plan of 290 carbohydrates. Although this was a fairly small change, Danny felt he'd been consulted, and mealtimes got a little easier.

Getting Organized

Even with nursing support, anxiety dogged both my husband and me. Now we had to pack a diabetes kit to leave the house. It contained insulin and syringes, alcohol wipes, a glucose meter and test strips, a juice box and snacks for lows, glucose oral gel to give Danny if he was too low to swallow, and a glucagon shot if he became unconscious. I also took any meals we might eat away from home. Caring for Danny required a lot of preparation and time for me to get used to all the new procedures. In those first weeks, I'd often be halfway somewhere before I realized I'd left some part of the kit at home. When you leave a diaper bag at home, all you risk is diaper failure and a mess. When you leave your emergency supplies at home…it's nerve-wracking.

At night, knowing that children with diabetes are at greatest risk of coma while they're sleeping, Brian and I kept a baby monitor by our bed. We'd been warned that a child could slip into a coma without ever waking up as his numbers dipped, so we got up and checked Danny in the middle of every night. Since I also knew that sometimes children with diabetes woke up and made sounds before they got too low, I found myself involuntarily waking up every time Danny rolled over or made noise. There is a sleep so light that in the morning you doubt that you ever closed your eyes. It was like having a new baby all over again, with no end in sight.

As the days passed, it was time to venture out and let Danny resume some of his normal activities. We had previously felt comfortable when the kids were away from us, trusting that they'd be okay. Now, however, I was nervous even when Danny and I were out together. What if I gave him the wrong dose of insulin? What if I lost track of time? What if we ran out of test strips, lancets or snacks? This was anxiety with a capital A, and all it took was a small glitch, like forgetting the test kit at home, to set my heart racing and my palms sweating. I also worried when Danny was with other people. What if they forgot to check him? Had I given them clear enough instructions? Had I told them about the juice box? Would they know to call 9-1-1 right away? The list went on and on.

I knew Brian was anxious too because he was calling home many times a day with similar questions. What were Danny's numbers? How much insulin was in his last dose? How did he seem? We put out more adrenaline in the first month than we'd used in the nineteen years we'd been together.

One way to allay that anxiety came to us loud and clear. Brian and I both got cell phones. I could now reach the doctor in an emergency. Danny could call me, no matter where I was or what I was doing. Everyone felt safer. As long as I stayed in places where the phone worked, help was only a phone call away. Brian kept his phone by his side. If he was in the office, his secretary knew that if I called with a problem, she should interrupt any meeting and find him. If he was out of the office, he left multiple numbers so I could reach him. We were on high alert and talked to each other by phone on and off all day.

Working as a Family Team

During those first few weeks, my husband took a lot of time off from work. Even though I was used to saying, "I can do it myself," when Brian decided he should stay home and help, I didn't argue. I was going through the motions well enough, but there were times when I was terrified. I would stand with an insulin shot in my hand and freeze. Had I double-checked the syringe to make sure there were no bubbles? Had I correctly calculated all the carbohydrates in Danny's snack? Did I know for sure that the old insulin was out of his body? Could this dose bring him too low?

Sometimes I would prepare a meal and end up lost in the cryptic pages of our carbohydrate counter. Did squash have the same number of carbohydrates as potatoes? How do you measure cheese sprinkled on spaghetti?

Brian's presence was a huge comfort, and when we were confused, we'd literally hunker down over the kitchen counter and look through diabetes books and our handouts. Sometimes, when I was frantically trying to reach our nurse at the hospital and listening to a never-ending stream of Muzak on the telephone, I would just lean against Brian and feel better.

During the first two weeks, incoming calls were a distraction we couldn't handle, and we let the machine take all our messages, answering only the crucial ones. This learning curve was the steepest we had ever encountered, and our single focus blotted out everything else. Diabetes became the topic of all of our conversation and suffused everything we thought, said, or did. Brian and I were completely dependent on each other, and our circle narrowed to the four of us.

By the end of two weeks, I'd mastered the daily routines enough so that life had a new rhythm, and Brian went back to work full-time. I could now care for Danny by myself, but having been so essential in the beginning, Brian continued to be in touch by phone during the day and attended the many doctors' appointments we had. Despite a lawyer's usual pressures, for several months Brian was home by six o'clock to help me with dinner, a drawn-out series of events that included meal preparation and a complicated medley of blood tests, phone calls to doctors, insulin calculations, and shots. Even with this support, I couldn't imagine finding the time or the peace of mind to counsel patients in my private practice. I extended my leave from work.

The kids were part of the team. One of the blessings of my life had been that I'd joined a mother's group when Danny was six months old. From this experience I had developed a mothering philosophy that went something like this: Everyone in a family has responsibility for helping things run smoothly, which means everyone has to do his or her share, tell the truth, not say or do anything hurtful on purpose, and apologize whenever that line is crossed.

This meant that by the time Danny got diabetes, my kids did their own laundry, helped unpack the dishwasher and the groceries, set and cleared the table, and pitched in when asked. As long as I didn't have to remind them, they could do most of these chores on their own schedule. If they grumbled too much or were mean to each other, I didn't get angry, but I added tasks. I explained, until they were sick of hearing it, that by fighting with each other or refusing to cooperate they were hurting the family and needed to make up for it. This meant folding more laundry or doing a sink full of dishes. If they argued, I added watering the plants or taking out the trash, which meant fewer chores for me. Unfortunately, they caught on quickly. Now, when I really needed their help, they were used to pitching in.

Jessie seemed to grow up overnight. She'd always been a typical oldest child, and often switched back and forth with Danny from playmate to mother hen. Now, at ten years old, she became astonishingly valuable. She paid close attention to all the details of his disease and often piped up with comments like, "He looks pale. Maybe you should test him," or "We should have meatballs because they have fewer carbohydrates." She was getting less attention than usual, yet whenever we asked how she was doing, she'd say, "Don't worry about me. I'm fine."

Everyone warned us not to leave her out of the loop, so we encouraged her to come to diabetes meetings and appointments. At times, it was tempting to send her to a friend's house or tell her to do her homework, but we kept her close to us and listened to her suggestions before we made decisions. We also arranged for her to spend time with friends and our extended family so she could get a break from the tension at home.

My mom asked her whether she was feeling left out and she said, "It bothers me sometimes that Danny gets so much attention. Whenever he's grumpy or tired, we don't know if he's low or not, so when he's acting like that, whatever we're doing, we stop. No matter what it is, Danny gets to sit down and relax. I know it's not Danny's fault, but it still bothers me. This might not be totally true, but it feels like he gets what he wants more than I do."

She was right. In the beginning, everything in our life did revolve around Danny's diabetes. All of us felt like his life was in our none-too-competent hands, so we tried to keep things as simple as possible. For the first month, we canceled all our activities, cleared our weekend schedule, and stayed home. We let the answering machine take our calls. We backed out of commitments at the kids' school, put off seeing friends, stopped working out, and only read books about diabetes. Our hands were full just keeping the family going. At the end of each day, Brian and I fell into bed at eleven thirty, too tired to talk, having set the alarm to wake us up in the middle of the night to test Danny's blood sugar again.

I felt as if each of us was the leg of a table, and that everyone had to do exactly what was needed to keep the table level. We were doing well as a team, but we were individually exhausted and overwhelmed. Diabetes had crowded out all the things that diverted or relaxed us, including kidding around. Giving Danny a shot was still very emotional for me, and with all the daily mini-crises, I couldn't seem to catch my breath.

I cannot imagine how we'd have survived that first month without the love and support of a huge network of people. My sister, Julie, who lives in the next town with her husband and two sons, brought us meals and welcomed Jessie warmly whenever she needed to get away. My mother-in-law, Anne, found out that her husband had cancer the same day that Danny was diagnosed, but she still found time to keep up a constant stream of calls and supportive e-mails. Brian's stepmother, Clara, immediately started reading diabetes books and became an extremely helpful person to talk to about the details. My parents' door was always open. Friends, family, and our Unitarian-Universalist church community brought meals.

The Juvenile Diabetes Research Foundation (JDRF) sent a representative who had a child with diabetes to tell us about available resources and invite us to a series of coffees.

The most disheartening thing she said was that it takes most families a whole year before they can do anything more than the bare minimum. It was also the most reassuring.

Preparing Friends and Teachers

It soon became clear that if Danny were going to continue visiting friends' houses, their parents had to understand diabetes and the basics of how to deal with it. One night we invited about fifteen neighbors and friends over and asked Robert, our visiting nurse, to give an introductory talk. Many compassionate and familiar faces surrounded me, but as I looked around, I felt vulnerable and raw. After welcoming them, my job was to explain that we needed them to watch over Danny when he was at their houses. I assumed I looked fine, but I was conscious of an invisible gulf between us.

"Please make sure he doesn't have snacks or candy without checking with us," I began. "If he looks tired or disoriented, call us. If he leaves your house to play outside, please have him call home so we can watch him." I couldn't banish the thought that their children could eat anything and go anywhere. Why would they want the responsibility of having Danny over? I was glad when my part was done.

Next Robert talked about the dangers. He explained that if Danny's sugars went under 80 (which is called hypoglycemia), his symptoms might be hunger, confusion, headache, tremors, clumsiness, stubbornness, or irritability. If he exhibited any of these, he should test his blood sugar and take glucose tablets, which would raise his numbers within ten minutes. Extreme hypoglycemia could result in collapse, seizures, or coma. If this happened, they should call 9-1-1.

As I listened to this scary narrative, I wondered what everyone was thinking. Should we have given them all this information? Would they still be willing to have Danny over? What was going to happen to Danny's friendships if the neighbors were afraid to take care of him?

I needn't have worried. My friends and neighbors may have been hesitant at first, but one successful visit led to another, and soon they were reassuring me that having my son over was no big deal. As time passed, too, Danny managed his own care with more independence and confidence. My fears that Danny's diabetes would disrupt his friendships turned out to be unfounded.

Before Danny returned to school, we set up a meeting with his teachers. There was no school nurse, so Mary, our VNA nutritionist, talked to the staff. She gave out the protocol on how to handle emergencies. Mary explained that if Danny's blood sugar went over 240 (which is called hyperglycemia), his symptoms might be dizziness, fatigue, irritability, confusion, hyperactivity, and behavior that appeared out of the ordinary. At these times, when blood sugar levels were too high, he needed more insulin. Unfortunately, she told everyone, highs feel like lows and look like them, too. That's why it's so important to test before acting.

Mary explained that if Danny was "high," he was supposed to drink water to dilute the sugar. Danny would have to go to the bathroom to urinate on a test strip and test for ketones (byproducts of fat metabolism in the urine when the blood is at a dangerous level of acidification). She demonstrated how to count carbohydrates at events like school birthdays and parties. Finally, she taught several brave souls how to give an emergency shot of glucagon, a hormone that makes the liver immediately release glucose into the bloodstream and raise blood sugar levels. I explained we'd send a lunch box full of food for Danny every day, with a list of what and when to eat.

I could see that the teachers clearly understood the gravity of the situation and were committed to helping Danny, but it was a lot to master in one sitting. At the end of the presentation, Danny's classroom teacher asked if I could stay at the school for a couple of days until everyone got comfortable with the changes. I was relieved and gladly accepted. I wasn't ready to leave Danny alone for long when his numbers were so unpredictable.

Every morning I went to school with Danny and stayed in the auditorium while he went about his day. I checked on him at ten in the morning and at noon. During the rest of the time, I tried to complete all the medical paperwork and mail-in pharmacy forms. Sometimes I read diabetes and nutrition books.

In those first weeks of January, our goal was to keep Danny's blood sugar numbers between 80 and 180. He tested either too low or too high at least once during every school day, and the teachers would come and ask me what to do. Then I would call the endocrinologist on call at the hospital for instructions. We couldn't get Danny's numbers regulated enough so that I could stay home. My stay stretched to five weeks, with no reassuringly normal days in sight.

One day I looked in on Danny through the window in his classroom door and noticed how lifeless he seemed. I interrupted the class. Danny had slipped into a passive state without telling anyone he was in trouble, and now he was so listless I had to hold his head up with my hands. I administered a blood glucose test; he was 38. I immediately opened a juice box, stuck the straw in his mouth, and prayed that he could drink. He did.

I'd been thinking that it was time to end my vigil, but now I asked myself, "What if I hadn't been there?" On the other hand, sitting in the school auditorium was making things worse. I had no one to talk to, and when someone did stop by, I found myself putting on false cheerfulness or choking up with tears. My life was full of unfinished tasks. I needed time to cook, shop, run errands, clean, see clients, and talk to my friends. I felt ready to disconnect, but I was scared.

I met with Danny's teachers at the end of that week, and to my relief, they said that they felt ready to handle everything. I couldn't protect Danny forever. At some point, I had to trust the world so I went home, mostly out of self-preservation. Luckily, this was the only time that he even came close to collapsing in school.

CHAPTER 3

▼

The First Three Months

The Importance of Educating Yourself

In my search for more information, I attended several Juvenile Diabetes Research Foundation coffees. All over the country, parents of children with diabetes gather in each other's homes for monthly meetings to meet each other and to discuss a specific topic or listen to a speaker. During my first coffee, it felt good to have things in common, to meet one another's eyes as we pulled out our cell phones and checked our signals before settling into the meeting. We all knew our children's morning blood sugar numbers and how many carbohydrates were in a bagel. We were all searching for trustworthy babysitters and trying to make a winning hand from the cards we'd been dealt.

I got some very practical advice. For example, several women told me that they didn't use alcohol swabs every time their children tested their blood; soap and water or a recent bath was clean enough. They also deemed it a waste of time and money to change the meter lancet before every test. I gave these women my full attention, determined to benefit from their experience. I met many people I liked a lot, who offered support and encouragement with an open heart.

I also read in all my spare moments, especially when I was sitting alone at Danny's school. I found helpful practical guides and diabetes Web sites on such topics as how to organize your pharmaceuticals, recognize and treat high and low blood sugars, travel, play sports, deal with schools, and handle sick days. I felt I was beginning to understand the medical issues underlying the disease.

I learned things our diabetes team hadn't told us. There was a new glucose meter called the Freestyle that would allow Danny to take a sample of blood from his forearm or calf instead of his sensitive fingertips. We could get smaller lancets to fit this meter, so that the pinpricks would be less painful. There were smaller syringes as well so that injections would hurt Danny less. I kept thinking, "What if I hadn't read this?" I soaked up information and took notes on ways we could improve what we were doing.

All the books I read shared one theme: Your child can do anything he or she wants to do, and everything is still possible. That sounded good to me because I wanted to encourage Danny to think of himself as a "normal" kid. Still, I had a nagging uneasiness about one aspect of the message. All the books supported letting your child eat whatever he wanted and insisted that cake, candy, and ice cream were okay. Let him have pizza, McDonald's, and Mexican food. You may have to increase the insulin, but whatever you do, don't let him feel deprived. That's what we'd been told at the hospital as well.

In addition, the diets in these books included many sugar-free products made with artificial sweeteners and colorings, as well as meat products with nitrates, such as beef jerky and bacon. These were recommended as foods that would fill Danny without requiring extra insulin. Yet, I had a child with an autoimmune disorder, and at some point, his body had been so stressed that his immune system had attacked the cells of his pancreas. Weren't we supposed to be improving his health in general? Shouldn't we do this by avoiding junk food and cutting back on sweets? Why wasn't I being told to avoid everything that might be hard for his body to process, like sugar-free products with unrecognizable ingredients? Then again, what did I know? Who was I to question the collective wisdom of the diabetes community?

I wavered back and forth on this issue, buying Danny sugar-free Jell-O one week and rejecting it the next. I'd like to say that Brian and I struck a happy medium between healthy eating and letting Danny "be a kid," but I had a series of mini inner struggles every time we made him a snack. The contents were either "too much like health food" or "too full of chemicals." I was critical of our choices either way.

By the end of the first month, I considered myself fairly well read on the subject of juvenile diabetes, and when my mother suggested that I read a book called *Dr. Bernstein's Diabetes Solution* by Richard K. Bernstein, M.D., I balked. I was craving escape.

"How about a romance novel?" I asked. She shook her head. She'd read this book and thought it was in the "must-read" category. I grudgingly took it from her, lugged it to Danny's school, and started in.

In the first chapter, Dr. Bernstein explains that he developed diabetes in 1946 when he was twelve. During the twenty-three years between his diagnosis and his first use of a blood glucose meter (not available until 1969), he did what children did at that time: he ate a high-carbohydrate, low-fat diet, testing his urine for blood sugar and giving himself one injection per day. By the age of thirty-five, he had high cholesterol, kidney stones, a stone in his salivary duct, "frozen" shoulders, impaired sensation in his feet, peripheral vascular disease that can lead to amputation, heart failure, failing vision, and advanced kidney disease. I read this section with a sense of doom. The long-term consequences of diabetes were lodging in my brain.

Then the story changed. Dr. Bernstein learned to monitor and regulate his blood sugar levels by using his new glucose meter. Through exercise and watching his diet, he started to feel better. In search of better health, he studied the effect of various foods on his glucose levels and developed a diet that kept his blood sugars at near-normal numbers around the clock. Eventually, most of his long-term complications disappeared. He once again felt robust and healthy.

I was eager to hear what he had discovered to be the ideal diet. It turned out to be extremely low in carbohydrates. Danny was currently on seventy-five carbohydrates at breakfast, eating pancakes or breakfast cereal and milk. Dr. Bernstein suggested eggs with breakfast meat or salmon with a bran cracker, only seven carbohydrates. Similarly, he suggested twelve carbohydrates at lunch and twelve at dinner. He explained that eating more carbohydrates and taking more insulin results in more errors and less predictability. Considering that Danny's numbers were jumping all over the place, I felt he had a point. He also said that instead of avoiding fat, children with diabetes should avoid carbohydrates, backing his assertions with documentation.

Having had little success convincing his doctors of the value of his approach, Dr. Bernstein became a doctor himself and opened a clinic where he helps people with diabetes attain near normal blood sugars without long-term complications. His success seemed astounding. After reading countless articles in which it was par for the course to have wide swings in blood sugar readings, here was someone who'd figured out how to make the numbers more predictable.

This book opened a window in my mind. I couldn't imagine limiting Danny to thirty-one carbohydrates per day, but there was a lot of room between thirty-one and his current regimen of 290. As I began reading books on nutrition, I discovered that Dr. Sears (the Zone Diet) and Dr. Atkins (the Atkins

Diet) believe that high levels of insulin may be a culprit in long-term health issues. They point out that for millions of years people ate what the earth provided: meat, vegetables, dairy, fruit, nuts, and seeds. Since this diet was necessarily low-carbohydrate, the pancreas only needed to provide small doses of insulin with each meal. Such ailments as diabetes, heart disease, and kidney failure are modern diseases linked to changes in our diet.

Danny would definitely need less insulin if he ate this way.

Then, I came across the term "glycemic index," which is a ranking of carbohydrates based on their immediate effect on blood glucose levels. The foods that break down quickly during digestion have higher indices, and the ones that release glucose gradually into the bloodstream have lower ones. Some researchers, I discovered, believe that ten carbohydrates of apple have a very different effect on the body than ten carbohydrates of grapes. Carrots, for example, have a high-glycemic index while nuts are low. These authors believe that strict adherence to foods low on the index can lead to better blood glucose control. Others stressed the importance of eating a wide variety of foods and questioned the validity of the glycemic index itself.

I'd assumed that there was only one way to approach and treat this disease: to test blood sugars, count carbohydrates, and give insulin. Now I had information that I hadn't seen in any of the diabetes books I'd read. Could low-carbohydrate meals be better for Danny? Would switching to foods with a low-glycemic index help us keep him steady? Why hadn't our doctors told us anything about this? Why hadn't anyone at the hospital mentioned a healthier diet during our three full days of educational meetings?

I kept reading. Our doctors had assured us that nothing we had done had caused Danny's diabetes and nothing we could do could cure it. Although no one on either side of our family had ever had Type 1 diabetes, they thought it was probably genetically linked and might have been triggered by a virus. Now I was reading articles by authors who thought diabetes in children might be linked to environmental toxins. I even received a call from a local woman who was mapping clusters of children with diabetes. She said that she was seeing patterns where several children in the same neighborhood were diagnosed with juvenile diabetes at the same time. My mother had read about a cluster close to an abandoned toxic dump near a local reservoir.

None of these claims could be satisfactorily substantiated, and the "why" of diabetes was something our family couldn't worry about, but I was once again reminded that I was not going to get the full picture from a brief visit to an endocrinologist every three months. Danny's well-being depended on my being well-informed.

In my reading, I kept coming across the term "honeymoon," which had been mentioned by Danny's doctors. This is a period of time after diagnosis when insulin needs decrease in some children. The theory is that after a child is put on insulin and his blood sugar is regulated, the pancreas is given a rest, enabling its beta cells to produce more insulin for several months. Since I firmly believed that Danny's own insulin would be better for him than the kind that came out of a vial, I wanted to know why he wasn't showing any signs of a honeymoon after four weeks of treatment.

I searched the Internet, books, and magazines that I had in the house. I couldn't find any information about how to precipitate the honeymoon. I wrote e-mails to the doctors and interns I'd met during our stay at the hospital, asking them how I could find out about research being done on this issue. I wrote to diabetes research centers in the United States, Germany, the Netherlands, and Israel. No one could tell me what stimulated the onset of the honeymoon, what prolonged the function of the islet cells during the honeymoon, or what caused it to end.

Finding Additional Care for Danny

Meanwhile we were distressed that Danny had started getting rashes, headaches, and stomachaches. We assumed these were side effects of the insulin or his roller coaster blood sugars, but our endocrinologist didn't think so. He referred us to our primary care physician who did blood work and a full physical exam. Dr. Horowitz could find no underlying cause, so we gave Danny Tylenol and Pepto Bismol. He continued to feel terrible. Brian and I wondered if Danny was under too much stress. There was certainly enough of it to go around. Many nights, while Danny lay awake in his bed, holding his stomach and crying, Brian and I felt completely helpless. Weren't we supposed to do something? We had talked to all his doctors. Where could we turn?

My parents were as worried as we were, and my father approached me with a suggestion. He had a friend who did "energy healing." Roland Baumgartel had once put his hands around my father's head for a few minutes and cured his headache. He'd helped people with the side effects of chemotherapy and the pain of arthritis. A construction supervisor by day, he saw people at night and on weekends, and because he felt the work was sacred, he refused to take any money for his time.

My dad offered to call him, but I had mixed feelings. What would Danny think of a man who healed with his hands? How could I accept help from someone I couldn't pay? All it took was one long afternoon of Danny lying on the couch, with his head in his hands and his knees drawn up to his chest, for me to change my tune. Within an hour, my father reported that Roland had volunteered to come to our house after work three times a week to see if he could help Danny feel better.

When Roland arrived the first time, Danny watched him warily. Roland was six feet, three inches tall and looked intimidating, even though his eyes were very kind. He explained to Danny that he had a gift for feeling the energy patterns that surround people's bodies. He could tell where they felt pain or where they needed help just by passing his hands four or five inches away from their clothing or skin. Sometimes, he said, he could then change the energy enough to help people feel better. He asked if he could spend five to ten minutes moving his hands around Danny's body without touching him.

Danny looked at me, shrugged, and said, "Sure." I'd been holding my breath, hoping he would accept a stranger's help, and now I sighed with relief. I was grateful to have found someone willing to do something.

As Danny stood in the living room fully clothed, Roland reported that he felt a heavy band of energy around Danny's abdomen, which he figured was a result of a digestive issue or problems with his pancreas. He also noted that he could feel heat under his arms and on the backs of his knees. Those areas were the location of Danny's rash, and neither Roland nor my father knew that. Perhaps, I thought, he knows what he's doing.

This was the first of many sessions. Each time Roland arrived, he'd begin by spending the first five or ten minutes running his hands over Danny's body during what he called the diagnostic phase. He had an uncanny ability to sense, without being told, if Danny had hurt his knee, been inactive, played computer games, or was especially tired. Then, for the next twenty minutes, Danny would lie on the couch, and Roland would concentrate on changing his energy into a healthier pattern by moving his hands back and forth over the areas that he felt needed work.

Sometimes Danny's headaches and stomachaches would completely go away, and we'd all be overjoyed. Sometimes they wouldn't, and Danny would ask why Roland had to come. Some days Danny's insulin needs would decrease or his rashes would go away, but the changes were temporary. It was hard for any of us to quantify how much Roland's visits helped.

Danny thought the process of lying still so long was boring, but he often fell into a deep sleep during the treatment and always seemed calmer afterwards. I found myself looking forward to Roland's visits because each time he arrived, he engaged me in conversation about Danny's symptoms, our doctors' appointments, and my current research. I was grateful that he brought an hour of comforting calm into our house and made me feel less alone.

Meanwhile, even though none of my diabetes books mentioned stomachaches, headaches, or rashes, my books on nutrition mentioned all of these symptoms. Some authors thought they were the result of food allergies while others thought that they were caused by large amounts of sugar, carbohydrates, food additives, or preservatives. Even though we didn't eat junk food, our picky eater rejected most fruits and vegetables and flatly refused any mixed foods like casseroles and soups. He favored white bread, French fries, fruit juice, and pasta. I wondered if I could change his diet without turning mealtimes into a battleground.

In order to minimize the changes in Danny's life, both the hospital and VNA nutritionists had matched his insulin dose to his preferred high-carbohydrate diet. He was now eating more carbohydrates and drinking more sugar-free products than before his illness. Both nutritionists had been so self-assured and professional that I hadn't questioned their assumption that we shouldn't fiddle with his usual diet.

Now, however, faced with Danny's symptoms, I started browsing through cookbooks looking for low-carbohydrate recipes that called for ingredients with low-glycemic indices. Dr. Bernstein's recipes seemed too austere, and the diabetes cookbooks I consulted favored complicated recipes that Danny was sure to reject, often suggesting artificial sweeteners or fat-free products filled with additives.

I was lost without a mentor.

God bless synchronicity! Within days, two acquaintances mentioned a woman named Deb Sawyer who'd helped their children overcome physical symptoms with nutritional advice and supplements. In February, one month after Danny's diagnosis, he and I drove two and one-half hours north to our first appointment. We both liked Deb immediately. She had done a lot of research on juvenile diabetes, and she recommended whole grain, high-protein, low-carbohydrate, organic meals with lots of vegetables. Treating Danny like an equal, she explained why a good diet was important and challenged him to enjoy a variety of foods.

Deb made specific recommendations based on her evaluation of Danny's food sensitivities. She prescribed a multivitamin and Chlorocaps, which provided the nutrients of green vegetables, since he refused to eat most of them. She put him on Primrose oil and acidophilus to help his digestion. Much to my amazement, he was willing to try some of the changes she recommended. When we returned home, he swallowed all those capsules without complaint.

Before we left, I described some of the symptoms of stress I was experiencing. I'd hit my shin on a stair and although the pain wasn't that bad, I'd had to sit down because I felt on the verge of fainting. At the hint of any difficulty, my heart would start to race as if there were a major crisis. I had periods when I couldn't fall asleep or slept so lightly that I didn't feel rested in the morning. Deb explained that after a trauma, adrenal glands often become overactive and then depleted. She suggested I take a supplement for adrenal support. I felt somewhat better within days of starting it.

At home, I started to make small changes in the food I served. I was already in the habit of putting out plates of cucumber, carrots, and celery with peanut butter before meals. The day after our visit to Deb, I replaced Skippy with an organic peanut butter. Danny tasted it and spit it out. The next day I hid the organic peanut butter underneath a thin layer of Skippy. He said it tasted delicious. After several days, I told him the truth and made him taste a stalk of celery filled with organic peanut butter. Reluctantly, he admitted that he liked it.

I started with baby steps. I replaced white bread with a commercial, relatively low-fiber whole-wheat loaf. The difference was a very slight change in color and a gram or two of fiber, and it took Danny about a week to get used to it. Then I bought natural oat bran bread the same color, but with a bit more fiber. It was two weeks before he stopped complaining. My goal became to move our whole family toward a healthier diet slowly without causing Danny too much distress. As his stomachaches, headaches, and rashes continued to come and go, he had enough to deal with.

Exercise

Every doctor, nurse, and author agreed on the positive impact of exercise. It strengthens the heart, stimulates the circulatory system, relieves stress, decreases the need for insulin, and most importantly, helps regulate blood sugars. Danny had always been an active kid, running around for long hours in the neighborhood, riding his bike, and playing soccer. Yet, even though we limited our children's television and computer use, on cold or rainy days he watched videos, played computer games at his friends' houses, or curled up and read a book.

Now we found that if Danny spent a Saturday morning on the couch, by lunch his blood sugar numbers were in the 300s. If we had to drive into the city for an appointment, which meant sitting in the car and the doctor's waiting room, he'd be high again. More than that, when we reacted by giving him higher doses of insulin, his numbers fell too low and Danny would feel weak, shaky, and sick. Brian and I were aware our decisions had caused his misery, so these roller coaster rides were terrible for everyone.

I struggled to keep Danny active. The kids and I would arrive home from a full day at their school, tired and stressed. I needed to clean up, return phone calls, and make dinner while Danny wanted to hang out, play Legos, or get his homework done. When we each did our own thing, his blood sugar levels were high by dinner and he felt terrible. I was distressed because I knew how his body was affected when his numbers rose too high. The long-term effects could be devastating.

That's why we sometimes found ourselves on a forced march, walking toward town in the late afternoon. My role was to make it into an adventure, Danny's to complain that he wanted to go home. Other times, even I would admit it was too cold or wet outside, and we'd go to the basement and make up obstacle courses or wrestle. We devised workout routines or challenged each other to see who could jump rope the longest. Sometimes Jessie joined us and that made the competition more intense and fast-paced.

After a while this extra exercise became a routine part of Danny's life, and he became aware that for the first time, he could run faster and longer than his peers. I loved how close it made us. We talked as we walked, and we laughed when we wrestled. It was a stress reliever for both of us. Nonetheless, with unopened mail stacked on the counter, the answering machine flashing madly, and the house near chaos, I relied on Brian to get Danny moving when he came home from work at night, and especially on the weekends.

Jujitsu is Brian's favorite hobby and his exercise. He's a black belt and he used to teach, but Danny's diabetes took its toll on that. He also belonged to a health club near his office and used to work out at lunchtime, but he gave that up completely when Danny was first diagnosed. He just couldn't find the time during the day to get his work done, talk to his clients, and go to the gym.

Now that he focused on getting Danny moving, he exercised at home. They put rubber mats on the floor in our basement where Danny and he made up as many games as possible. They played a game called "Kill Ball," where the idea was to throw a big soft playground ball into a square area on the wall while the defensive player tries to prevent the goal by stopping the ball with his body. They invented a game they called "Gladiator," where they wore foam protective gear and hit each other with big foam clubs. Since Brian was on the wrestling team in high school, they wrestled. They also played floor hockey and basketball with small hoop sets at each end of the room.

Outside when the weather was nice, Brian and Danny played lacrosse, basketball, soccer, and catch with every imaginable ball and frisbee. Brian made up a game called "Tenny Square," a combination of four-square, volleyball, tennis, and ping-pong, which they played with a playground ball on a court chalked on the street. When the small pond across the street was frozen, they ice-skated and played ice hockey on the lighted surface in the evenings. Considering how many adjustments Brian had to make, he found that he wasn't in bad shape.

A Close Call with My Mother

My mother's first attempt to take my kids somewhere was a near disaster. She decided that she couldn't let her fear of messing up interrupt their relationship so she made plans for a short trip to the Museum of Science. Danny, Jessie, and my mother would drive in at ten o'clock in the morning, see a one-hour IMAX movie, get Danny's blood sugar reading, follow my chart for how much insulin to use, and give him his shot. They'd eat lunch at the museum where Danny could order chicken and fruit. Then they'd come home.

It would take only four hours. My mother felt she could do this, especially since Jessie had been paying close attention to every shot, every meal, and every dinnertime crisis. Having Jessie there made my mother feel safer.

They were within sight of the Museum of Science when they began to smell a burning, bitter odor. While they were looking around to see if something was burning outside, a thick black cloud of smoke rose up from under the hood of my mother's 1984 station wagon. The kids panicked.

"The car's on fire," Jessie shouted. My mother quickly pulled over into the parking lot of a rehabilitation hospital, urged the kids out of the car, pulled out the key, and jumped out herself. Her dog Pandora, who had come along for the ride, followed the children. With the engine off, the car settled into a grim silence.

The Museum of Science was out. Now they needed to find a way home. My mother went into the hospital, sat the kids against the wall, and used a pay phone to call Brian. He'd come into the city by train and didn't have his car. She called some friends who weren't home. Since dogs aren't allowed on the subway, she finally called AAA, and prayed that the mechanic would be willing to tow them all to a garage near home.

She tucked Pandora back in the car while Jessie and Danny sat down on a curb in the hospital parking lot. It was only eleven thirty, not yet time to worry about Danny's insulin. Finally, the tow truck arrived. The driver was explaining that he'd be breaking the law if he towed a car with a dog in it, when my mother noticed that Danny was crying. He'd been very quiet and good, waiting patiently until then.

"I'll be right back," she told the tow truck driver and went over to Danny.

"I know it's tough to be disappointed like this, but as soon as the car is fixed, we'll come back to the Museum of Science," she told Danny. "Don't be sad."

He nodded, but tears kept trickling down his cheek.

"Nana," Jessie said hesitantly. "I think he's low."

My mother's throat tightened. It was only eleven thirty in the morning. She wasn't supposed to check yet, but she could see that Danny's eyes had a strange faraway look. She tested Danny's blood sugar; he was 43. If Jessie hadn't caught him in time, he might have become unconscious. His patience hadn't been patience at all. He'd been disoriented, passive, and overwhelmed by his body's reaction. Meanwhile, my mother couldn't remember how to work the glucagon shot. Still, she panicked and grabbed for the red case in Danny's pack.

"Don't give him glucagon, Nana," Jessie said, "or he'll have to go to the hospital. We should try the tube of frosting first." My mother emptied the tube into Danny's mouth and had Jessie stay next to him, promising to call out if she noticed him getting worse. She headed back to the tow truck driver.

"My grandson's reading was just too low," she explained, her heart pounding, her hands trembling. "He's just been diagnosed with diabetes, and I don't know what I'm doing. I can't just abandon the dog, and I can't even think. I don't know what to do." The driver looked from her to the kids. Jessie had her arm around Danny's shoulders.

"If I put the dog in my cab," he asked, "will it stay on the floor?"

My mom threw her arms around him. "Thank you, thank you," she whispered. "Come on, kids. We're going home."

Danny was able to walk to the truck without much trouble. His eyes were brighter; he was returning to himself. They crowded into the cab, a tight fit for four across. Pandy lay at their feet. Danny and Jessie explained to the driver what had just happened. He listened sympathetically, and it began to sound like an adventure. Their car had blown up. They were evading the law, smuggling the dog home under the eyes of the traffic police. They were riding, squashed together, in the cab of a big tow truck. The dog had stranded them in an impossible situation, and they'd triumphed just the same. They agreed it made a great story.

Their new friend dropped the car off at my mother's garage and drove them right to my front door. After the kids told me their amazing story, my mother went home, threw herself into bed, and cried. Later she called me and sounded very upset.

"Laura, I almost hurt Danny. I wasn't attentive enough. I couldn't recognize an insulin low when I saw one. If it hadn't been for Jessie and the kindness of a stranger, our 'story' might have been a tragedy. I let you down. The frosting tube slipped my mind. I couldn't have used the glucagon shot if I'd had to."

I tried to reassure her, but she continued. "I'm angry with myself. I've been in bed all afternoon, not answering the phone, thinking of everything I did wrong. But," she paused, "I'm getting up now."

There was a long silent moment, and then she sounded better. "This is what's important. You need me and no matter how sorry an excuse for a grandmother I am, I'll learn what I need to know. I'll do better next time. I love you with all my heart and I'm not going to chicken out."

I had been home all afternoon blaming myself. I'd felt that if there was anyone that I could trust to handle Danny, it was my mother, but she had obviously needed more support. I should have sent an emergency sheet, a primer on what do in every situation. Why hadn't we reviewed the safety information and the glucagon shot procedure before she left? I reassured my mother that we would work together to figure it all out, and she got off the phone with new resolve. Neither of us dreamed that within a year, she and Danny would spend a whole day at the Museum of Science without a moment's concern.

My first priority was telling Jessie how grateful I was that she had been calm and capable in a crisis.

A Breakthrough with Acupuncture

The unpredictability of Danny's numbers remained mystifying. With the same amount of insulin and the same number of carbohydrates at breakfast, he could be 68 at lunch one day and 281 the next. He received two to three shots a day, and we recorded blood sugars that ranged from a low of 37 to a high of 440. Although we carefully calculated and monitored his meals, it seemed impossible to attain any stability in his readings.

His numbers set me off on an emotional roller coaster. I raced from relief to bitter disappointment in the time it took to read the meter while trying to project a feeling of calm detachment. The meter might say 360 and I might be thinking, "Oh no, I have to call the hospital again," but I'd shrug and tell Danny, "Well, we'll get better at this." He continued to have headaches, stomachaches, and rashes. There was no sign of the honeymoon.

Brian and I found it impossible to stand by idly when our child didn't feel well most of the time. We wanted do something. My friend Annie had been diagnosed with stage three breast cancer four years earlier and had chosen surgery and acupuncture instead of chemotherapy and radiation. She was now in remission as far as the doctors could tell, and she felt that her Korean acupuncturist had saved her life. She encouraged me to call him and ask if he'd ever treated children with diabetes.

The staff at the New Life Health Center said that Bo-In Lee, Lic. Ac., had never treated children with Type 1 diabetes, but had had considerable success getting Type 2 diabetes patients off insulin and helping with long-term complications. The receptionist gave me the names of several people he'd treated. I made phone calls to confirm the success of acupuncture in these cases, and then made an appointment for a consultation at the end of February.

When Brian and I took Danny to Bo-In Lee the first time, he explained his use of acupuncture needles, customized herbal formulas, breathing techniques, and therapeutic exercises resembling yoga. He shared his belief that diabetes is caused by an imbalance of the organs and energies in the body and said that his goal would be to create balance and let the body heal itself. Instead of believing that the honeymoon was something that occurred by chance, he thought he could start it and reduce Danny's need for insulin right away. I wasn't sure I'd heard him correctly. Had I really found someone who not only thought the honeymoon was worth pursuing, but felt he could trigger it?

His next words cut through my reflections. "In Korea we find that children sometimes have a very long honeymoon. When you have a balanced body, you can stop the immune system from attacking itself and prolong the life of the islet cells." Then he turned to Danny. "You have to make big changes, though. You have to eat lots of vegetables and nothing white—no dairy, no white sugar, no white flour. You have to exercise every day and get your heart going." He got up and walked vigorously around the room with his arms pumping at his sides. When he returned to his seat, he continued, "You have to breathe deeply into your stomach. You have to do yoga and relax."

I was still back on the words, "stop the immune system." Was it possible? Had it ever been done? I realized Bo-In Lee was waiting for a response from Danny. Was he willing to make changes? Surprisingly, my son was nodding his head. He was willing to exercise. He would try to like more vegetables. Then he tilted his head and asked, "What's yoga?"

Bo-In Lee smiled and rose from his chair. "You will see, my good boy. I will show you after you are used to the acupuncture."

We entered the treatment room, and Bo-In Lee put one needle in Danny's arm. "It doesn't hurt," Danny reported.

"Good, good," said Bo-In Lee and removed it. "That is your first treatment. We will see you next week and you will have more needles. It is good to start slow."

Somewhat dazed, Brian, Danny, and I walked to the car. We'd come with the hope that he could get some physical relief from his symptoms. We hadn't expected Bo-In Lee to make dramatic changes. Nowhere in any of my reading had anyone mentioned the possibility of inducing the honeymoon or slowing down the progression of the disease. Then again, no one had asked us to make drastic changes in Danny's diet.

We were excited, but the treatments were expensive and the drive was an hour each way through city traffic. These things felt overwhelming. We talked in the car all the way home, and by the end of the ride we'd come to an agreement. Danny would continue to make small changes to his diet, and he'd try six sessions. If nothing changed, we'd stop the treatments.

The only thing we had to lose was a tiny twinge of hope.

On the first Wednesday in March, Danny got his first full treatment. I went with him and watched as he lay on a paper-covered table under a heat lamp while Bo-In Lee inserted a series of tiny child-size needles into his abdomen, arms, legs, feet, and hands. Some of the needles were painless, and some, Danny reported, tears silently dripping from his eyes, really hurt.

I felt sick to my stomach. I was filled with doubts. If acupuncture didn't work, would Danny resent our having put him through this? Were we taking advantage of a seven-year-old child's desire to please his worried parents? Was a gamble worth his pain? To my astonishment, my son didn't resist or attempt to get up from the table.

Bo-In Lee was firm, but extremely kind and reassuring, saying, "What a brave boy you are. What a good boy. You are stronger than some of the adults I treat."

Looking back, I think Danny acquiesced because he wanted to feel better, but during that first treatment I felt ill. We left with a bottle of herbal pills to support Danny's pancreas.

On the drive home, Danny told me that he was feeling low. We tested his blood sugar, and he was right. He drank some juice to bring himself back into a normal range. This was the first in a series of lows that afternoon and early evening. Brian and I exchanged meaningful looks as we decided to decrease the number of units we gave him in his bedtime shot.

I was purposefully matter-of-fact with Danny all week as his need for insulin dropped lower and lower. He came home from school each day reporting lows at snack and lunch, and each morning we dropped his dose. I was careful not to react in any way, though inside me hope was bubbling up like soda that has been shaken in a can. I didn't want Danny to care about the numbers, and Brian and I never talked about what seemed to be happening. I think we were afraid we would jinx the outcome.

The day before his first acupuncture treatment, Danny had had three shots and a total of fifteen units of insulin. A week after the treatment, he was on one shot of six units!

Research has shown that a reduced need for insulin usually begins spontaneously soon after diagnosis, but it was two months into Danny's illness and immediately after his first acupuncture treatment that he started his honeymoon. We were convinced the acupuncture made the difference.

By the time Danny leveled off at six units, he was making enough insulin so that he didn't need a shot during the night. We shut off the baby monitor and enjoyed nights of blissful, unbroken sleep. We continued to test his blood sugar levels at breakfast, lunch, dinner, and bedtime, but the only time he needed a shot was first thing in the morning. One of the best changes was that his headaches, rashes, and stomachaches disappeared. Our life seemed less pressured and less medical. Whether he felt better because of the acupuncture or Roland's energy treatments or healthier food or the decrease in insulin, we didn't care. All we knew was that Danny was full of energy again.

Finally, we allowed ourselves to feel elated.

I took Danny to two more acupuncture visits and his insulin needs stayed low. At our fourth appointment, Bo-In Lee mentioned that he thought we should stay for a week at his clinic. During that week, Danny would get daily treatments and together we could practice yoga, eat specially prepared foods, and attend lectures on nutrition and lifestyle changes.

The cost was high and it was not covered by insurance, but we had the money in savings. Brian and I decided that Danny and I should go and I was excited by the prospect, but when I told Danny, I got a glimpse of something unexpected.

Danny's never been one to like changes, so I was expecting resistance. When he said he didn't want to go, I countered with this argument, "Danny, there's a very small chance that you can do without insulin for a while, and we think it's worth making the best of this opportunity."

Looking up at me from an elaborate Lego construction, he remarked in all seriousness, "I don't mind it."

"What do you mean?"

"I don't mind having diabetes. I've *only* had it for two months."

He said it in a plaintive way, as if I were threatening to take away a gift he'd just gotten. Brian and I would have done anything to find a cure for this illness, yet Danny didn't seem anxious to give it up. How could he be so matter-of-fact about an event that had turned our lives upside down?

Then it hit me. As a second child, Danny was now the center of an enormous amount of loving attention. We were revolving around him, not his sister. Also, he didn't know a thing about the possible consequences of his disease. We hadn't mentioned them to either of the children. My husband had always answered Danny's question, "Am I sick?" with "No, you're not sick. You can do everything you've always done. It's just that you have a medical condition."

Danny trusted us completely, and now he also had a sense of well-being. In the end, I got him to Bo-In Lee's by reassuring him that even if he went off insulin, we'd have to watch him very, very closely.

I told my mother about Danny's reaction. She told me what he'd said when she asked him how his life was different since he'd been diagnosed. He answered, "The only thing that's different is the eating. I can play soccer, I can swim, and I can do anything I could before. I don't mind it."

Who knew?

A Visit to the Emergency Room

Toward the end of March, Brian's brother Duffy came to stay with us for a while after returning from a trip to Mali, West Africa. The next day he fell ill from a stomach flu he must have contracted there. Brian and I fell asleep praying that our son wouldn't catch it, but the next night Danny started throwing up too. On the morning of his eighth birthday, he couldn't hold anything down.

At the endocrinologist's advice, we gave Danny his usual amount of insulin and then tried to get him to drink juice and eat Popsicles to keep hydrated. He lay on the couch, desperately sad to be missing his own, much-anticipated birthday party at school. Often stomach flu can be handled comfortably at home, but after Danny tested positive for ketones, I had to tell him that he would be spending his birthday in the hospital. Our family doctor called a local hospital emergency room, and they said we should bring him right in.

Danny was so weak that he couldn't walk and so heavy that I couldn't carry him. I stood in the middle of the living room trying not to panic. Since he'd taken in almost nothing, I was scared he'd have a hypoglycemic episode on the way to the hospital. I called my parents, and the two of them helped me get Danny into the car.

When we got to our local hospital, all twenty-one cubicles in the emergency room were filled and, although we told the triage nurse about our situation, we sat for hours without attention. Even though the staff had been alerted to the fact that Danny had diabetes, no one tested his sugars or asked us what they were. Despite our frequent pleas, we couldn't get anyone to look at him. My mind couldn't make sense of it. My child's head was drooping. Where were the doctors, the nurses, the IVs? We were in a hospital, yet his life remained in my hands. I tried to ward off dehydration by giving Danny apple juice while we waited, but he could barely take a sip.

When I couldn't stand it any longer, I paced. I'd go to the nurses' station. Most times no one was there, but on a few occasions, someone behind the counter would look up. I tried to be polite as I told them Danny was looking worse and worse, and they assured me every time that it would soon be our turn. I wanted to yell, but the nurses were so overwhelmed and the emergency ward so understaffed, there was no one to yell at. Even my dad, pulling rank as a doctor, couldn't get anyone to respond.

By the time we had a cubicle, the two nurses who came to give Danny an IV couldn't find a vein, no matter how many times they stuck him. We had to wait for them to find a specialist to insert the IV. It took this harried woman quite a few sticks before she succeeded. Danny didn't protest; he just sobbed silently throughout the whole procedure.

Once the IV needle was in, we waited in the cubicle another half-hour for the actual IV machine to arrive. After it was connected, we heaved a sigh of relief. Danny lay with his eyes closed for five minutes before we realized the nurse had failed to plug in the machine. We summoned a second nurse who plugged the machine in, but failed to get the fluid flowing, so we had to call her back. It took five hours before Danny was treated.

After the IV started dripping, Danny perked up. He opened our birthday gift, and my mother took a photo of him smiling in his white hospital robe. Since we couldn't invite anyone over for his birthday because he was contagious, we promised him a party the next weekend. He quietly took in the news and then turned his head away so I couldn't see his face. An hour later, Danny's nausea had subsided and we were free to go home.

Posttraumatic Stress

Although Danny was recovering, I felt numb. I was aware of ignoring feelings just below the surface, but I just kept going. One morning, a few days after our ER visit, I woke up crying uncontrollably. I tried to get up, but if the kids saw me, they'd worry and I didn't want to explain that I felt as if the world was caving in on us. I was afraid the next phone call would bring bad news, the next knock at the door another accident, the next morning another illness. Life seemed overwhelmingly fragile and frightening. I dreaded getting out of bed.

After Brian left for work, I climbed into the shower. I sobbed, letting the stream of water drown out the sounds coming out of me. I don't know how long I stood there, but eventually I felt better. The pain was still there, but most of the energy had leaked out of it. I went downstairs. Danny was watching television. He needed a shot and I was the only one able to estimate how much insulin he needed, so I pulled myself together. Soon the rhythm of the day swept me up, and I stopped thinking about anything but my next task.

A few days later, I was browsing on the Internet when I came upon a brief report on posttraumatic stress disorder in parents of children with newly diagnosed Type 1 diabetes, which put my experience in a new light. Researchers had studied the parents of thirty-eight children with newly diagnosed Type 1 diabetes by giving them the Post Traumatic Diagnostic Scale six weeks after diagnosis. They found that 24 percent of the mothers and 22 percent of the fathers met full diagnostic criteria for current PTSD. In addition, 51 percent of the mothers and 43 percent of the fathers met criteria for partial PTSD. The age and gender of the child, socioeconomic status, family structure, or length of hospital stay didn't seem to make a difference.

So I wasn't the only one finding this stressful. These last few months had affected me physically, no question about it. I'd been in a constant state of hyper-vigilance since the day Danny got hit by the car, and it only intensified when he fell off the skateboard and loosened his teeth. Obviously, it got worse when he was diagnosed. The impact had been cumulative.

I felt in the middle of a crisis even when there was no emergency. I had an involuntary sinking feeling in my stomach every time Danny's numbers ran high. I had periods when I woke at night or in the early morning and couldn't fall asleep again because my mind was racing. I became so used to feeling tired and anxious, I could barely remember the moments of well-being that used to punctuate my days. In addition, my neck and back problems returned even though I'd been pain-free for ten years.

Was this posttraumatic stress? Was this happening to almost half of us?

In these first months, I turned to my parents more than at any other time in my adult life, and I discovered that my mother was struggling with her own emotions as well. It's clear that there are wonderful things about living near us. She and my father get to be part of what's happening and to share the joys of the next generation. However, there are some terrible things about it too. They get to see the sorrows firsthand, and after Danny's diagnosis, life seemed to consist of one crisis after another.

One day over coffee, my mother explained her feelings. "Knowing what's going on allows me to help, but it resembles the worst parts of parenthood all over again. I worry that worry will swallow me up and absorb all my energy. I'm struggling to find a way to keep a peaceful and sane distance from everything going on."

I asked her if she needed some time off and some distance from the whole situation, but she shook her head. "No, it's not that. I recognize, deep in my gut, that you don't 'need' a mother anymore. Whatever you haven't absorbed growing up in our house, you aren't going to learn from me now. Whenever I feel tempted to rescue you, I remind myself that you're a grown woman and that you and Brian can take care of yourselves and your children. It's your job to worry. It's my job to be there when you need me, no matter what happens, no matter how I feel."

I suggested that I stop telling her as much, but she waved that thought away. "Most of the things I brood about are products of my imagination anyway. When I feel myself getting anxious, I take a deep breath, call upon my will and my intention and calm myself. It helps to remind myself that I don't need to add my distress to an already distressing situation."

Soon after this conversation, we found a new way to be together. When I stopped by her place, wanting to talk, my mother sat down at her computer and wrote down my words. She is a writer, and the process turned out to be therapeutic for both of us. She found her mind quieting as she concentrated on following my train of thought, and somehow putting my concerns into her computer kept her from feeling we were merging. In some ways, this became a spiritual exercise. It was as if we were both taking the time to consecrate this new reality, which had come unbidden and had to be accepted. Somehow, she was able to leave her worries behind when she put her computer to sleep, and I left feeling lighter, too.

My mother has concluded that she has one main contribution to make to my family—to love us. "That means keeping my eye on where the real needs are. That means becoming a rock when the waves crash in full force. That kind of love is keeping me sane while I watch every last one of Danny's insulin-producing cells die, one by one, knowing that there's nothing on God's earth I can do to change it."

CHAPTER 4

▼

The Second Three Months

Getting Away Overnight as a Couple

My parents offered to take both kids overnight at the beginning of April. Brian and I were hesitant to leave them, but diabetes had taken the place of all the things we used to talk about and we badly wanted some uninterrupted time together. Danny was recognizing his lows before they got dangerous, and he seemed to have a good understanding of his illness. So we said yes.

According to my mother, it was a comedy of errors. My father and mother agreed to take both kids Saturday afternoon, keep them overnight, bring them to church, and then entertain them until early Sunday evening. Since Danny tested his own blood sugar levels, knew what he could and couldn't eat, and could give himself his own shots, they felt confident. I wrote out a schedule that covered every contingency I could think of.

My mom was apologetic when she met us at the door on Sunday.

"I knew somewhere in my brain that Danny needed exercise every day, but I forgot. We spent Saturday afternoon watching a movie. As a result, Danny mostly sat around, and his blood sugar levels rose. At church the next morning, I got busy talking to friends and didn't keep an eye on what Danny was eating during coffee hour. While I assumed he could be trusted, he was snacking on pastry. I can't resist anything sweet if it's put on the table in front of me. Why did I assume Danny had more willpower than I do? At age eight, how could he say 'no' to cookies when everyone else was eating them?"

Then my dad chimed in with his description of Sunday's lunch.

"I'd planned to take Danny to a Thai restaurant where Danny knew exactly what to order, but Danny wanted to go Mexican. When he assured me nachos were fine, I didn't bother to consult his carbohydrate counter. We shared the nachos, and I figured he'd gotten some protein. His blood sugar before lunch was 138, but by three that afternoon, even with insulin, it was 350."

Brian and I were up all night trying to get his numbers down. As we talked about it, my parents decided they'd relied too much upon Danny. Despite how much responsibility he took for his illness, he was just eight years old. They also said they fell into the habit of getting on with life as usual and forgot that Danny had different, very specific needs. My dad realized, sort of, that he needed to be less cavalier.

"You've been so conscientious that there have been very few situations where I've had to make decisions about Danny's care. I've allowed myself to enjoy him without thinking about myself as a potential source of help or information. I know there's a downside to my attitude, yet I can't help but think my biggest contribution is to maintain for myself and for Danny the happy fiction that everything is fine."

Even though Danny's numbers were high and my parents were tired, the kids had a great time, and Brian and I enjoyed the break. We slept through most of it, but when we were awake, we focused on each other and put our worries aside. It may not have worked out perfectly for Danny, but it felt vital for us.

Trying to Balance the Demands of Work and Home

Three months after diagnosis, we received Danny's first Hemoglobin A1c report, a value that represents his average blood sugar level for the preceding three months. A normal person's range is between four and six. Studies show that Hemoglobin A1c's over eight are correlated with a higher incidence of serious long-term complications, such as kidney failure, heart disease, and circulatory problems leading to amputation, impotence, and blindness. Some of Dr. Bernstein's patients were reportedly in the four to six ranges, but children's numbers can go as high as twelve or thirteen if they aren't conscientious about caring for themselves.

Danny's number was 7.2. Brian and I were surprised it was that low. The doctor assured us that everything was fine, and we nodded and moved on.

At this point, taking care of Danny was a full-time job. To provide three meals and four snacks took an enormous amount of planning, shopping, and preparation.

Every day I made sure Danny exercised, and I spent hours reading books and researching diabetes and nutrition on the Internet. I maintained contact with his teacher, trained babysitters, and talked with the parents of Danny's friends every time he went to a friend's house. Once a week I picked him up after school, and we went to acupuncture and out to dinner. Roland still came once a week to do energy healing. I was calling endocrinologists and seemed to live at the pharmacy. We also had regular appointments with our nutritionist and our nurse diabetes educator.

Meanwhile, I was trying to be the same wife, mother, and friend I'd always been, but my friends were being crowded out of my life. I was spending so much time on the phone with medical personnel, pharmacies, and our insurance company that at night the last thing I wanted to do was call someone and chat. I didn't see friends in the evening because I didn't feel it was fair to leave Brian alone with all the bedtime decisions. Occasionally I'd stop by someone's house in the morning after I dropped both kids off at school, and some of my friends started stopping by at random times, knowing I was usually in the kitchen.

I went to school conferences, kept dentist appointments, went shopping for clothes with Jessie, and returned videos and library books. I cleaned house and ran all the errands it takes to keep a household with two children going. There already weren't enough hours in the day, yet for some reason I don't fully understand, I felt an internal pressure to go back to work.

I'd stopped working part-time as a counselor in January. When Danny was diagnosed, I called my clients and told them that it would take me several months to adjust to our new family situation. Many of these clients took my suggested referrals and found new therapists, but some decided to wait for me. Thankfully, Brian's salary was enough to support us, and we agreed that I should stay home until I felt ready.

Ready or not, I began seeing a few clients on Wednesday mornings. The excitement of being a professional adult again carried me through my early sessions. I was thrilled to be back and eager to prove to myself that I could resume my life as a working mother. I had missed my clients and was happy to have them back in my life.

At first, the difficulty of resuming work one morning a week seemed like a matter of settling down. When I sat across from someone at the beginning of a session, I'd notice troubling worries in my head: *Is my cell phone on? Did I set it to vibrate or ring? Is my battery charged enough to last through this hour?*

"Danny's fine," I'd remind myself. "Pay attention to what's happening here." Sometime later, the phone in the office I shared with another therapist would invariably ring. I'd try to ignore it. Then I'd think, *Is someone trying to reach me about Danny? Is someone calling me at the office instead of on my cell phone?*

"Nothing bad is happening," I'd reassure myself. "Relax and be present." If the phone rang again, I'd break out in a light sweat and count the minutes until the session was over, so I could check the answering machine. I'd never felt any level of anxiety at work before, and I kept hoping my nervousness would go away as I adjusted to my new routine.

Finally, I had a very bad day.

I was sitting with a client who was telling me how tired she was because her kids had awakened her early. *Well, at least you were sure they were going to wake up,* I thought. She started complaining about how difficult her son's birthday party had been because her husband refused to help. *At least your son didn't sit in the ER on his birthday while you were terrified he might die,* I said to myself. She said she was overwhelmed. I tried to push away the thought, *you have no idea what overwhelmed means.* I was used to having a very attentive mind while I worked. I didn't compare my patients' lives to mine or judge the seriousness of their problems. At least I hadn't before this.

Now I could barely listen.

I'd changed, maybe not forever, but at least for now. I was distracted by my own problems and anxious when I was out of touch; it took an enormous amount of effort to hide it. More importantly, I was struggling to make sense of what was happening to our family. I didn't have the resources to spend hours focusing on other people's concerns. To be honest, I wished I were the one sitting on a couch with someone listening patiently to me.

Soon after, I told my clients I'd be taking an indefinite leave.

Brian had to make major changes in his life as well. He adjusted his work hours to meet Danny's needs. Mealtimes were particularly difficult so he began going into work after preparing breakfast and coming home before dinner. He took time out during the day to attend all the doctors' visits, which initially were as frequent as every two weeks, and to attend meetings with nutritionists, visiting nurses, and teachers.

He went to appointments with me because managing juvenile diabetes is an extremely thought-intensive process. Blood sugar levels are always bouncing around and the responses to food, insulin, and exercise are inconsistent, so it took a lot of concerted effort every time we planned a meal together or assessed Danny's dose. That process is easier when you can talk it over. This way neither of us had the sole responsibility for making decisions.

We made a big effort to have as equal a share of the diabetes management as was possible. Every day when Brian got home, he checked Danny's chart. We were always talking about his blood sugars, what they meant, how best to control them, and whether we should be changing things. Brian knew it wasn't easy for me to be alone on the front line, so he called me from work two or three times a day and always took my call if I phoned the office.

Brian also changed the way he worked. He intentionally cut out many extras, like continuing education and client development. He eliminated evening events, such as taking clients to ball games, having drinks after work with them, and going to cocktail parties where he might meet new people. He no longer took the time to go to seminars since he needed that time in the office to get his work done.

Brian brought more work home and would do work on the train or after we got the kids into bed. In the office, he tried to focus on the most important things to do. He delegated a lot of work to associates while he spent his time returning phone calls and answering his clients' questions. This way he could give his clients more personalized attention. He was moving in that direction anyway, but Danny's illness helped him prioritize. It was fortunate that he'd chosen to leave several fairly rigid law firms earlier in his career and had found a good and understanding partnership. The result was that his partners and associates were sympathetic, and there was never any criticism of his reduced hours. Luckily, he'd also hired good people to assist him.

Danny's Honeymoon: Off Insulin!

On the second Monday in April, Danny and I left for our week at the acupuncture center. It was both fun and difficult. Danny said the treatments were painful, the yoga was boring, and the simple Korean meals were too healthy, but he loved going on daily afternoon outings with me to the Franklin Park Zoo and the Arnold Arboretum and having so much time together. He also felt very close to Bo-In Lee, who hugged and patted him on the head at every opportunity, calling him a "good boy," with obvious affection. After one particularly difficult session, Bo-In Lee gave Danny a ten-dollar bill and sent us skipping to the local toy store. Danny trusted him and became more and more committed to doing whatever he could to get better. We saw results immediately. By the end of the week, Danny was receiving only two units of insulin once a day.

During the week, I walked an emotional tightrope. I was feeling hopeful and excited as I watched Danny's numbers fall and his need for insulin decrease. I felt relaxed since the risk of severe lows had diminished. Bo-In Lee was getting the results he had predicted, and our days were getting easier. We were sleeping through the night and Danny's numbers predictably fell between 80 and 110 in the morning. At the same time, I was aware that at any moment the treatments could stop working.

The endocrinology team at the hospital was continually warning our family about the dangers of "false hope," saying that any honeymoon period would be short-lived since *no* child had ever been cured of juvenile diabetes. They assured us that many children temporarily reduce their need for insulin in the first few months, but the remaining islet cells always succumb to the unceasing attack of a destructive immune system eventually. Our team had never treated a child who received acupuncture treatments; they believed the start of the honeymoon was a coincidence.

At the clinic, I tried to stay away from value judgments. I didn't want either of us to despair if Danny's numbers started to rise again. If Danny's numbers were low, even after a large meal, I'd say, "Wow your pancreas is making an awful lot of insulin. Let's give you less in your shot tomorrow." If they were toward the high side, I might say, "Good thing we gave you your shot this morning. It's helping you stay in range."

He never asked, "Am I going to go off insulin?" and I never said I wanted him to, but sometimes we'd look at each other with conspiratorial smiles, and I knew that thought was in both our minds. Inside, I felt like I was witnessing a miracle. Even if it didn't last another day, Danny and I had this one.

When we got home, we continued with the supplements, with Roland's energy healing sessions, and with weekly acupuncture visits. I continued to change our family's eating habits one at a time: more fruit, vegetables, meat, nuts, and good fats—less bread, pasta, rice, potatoes, and sugar. We gradually reduced our carbohydrate intake. Danny went from 335 to 290 to 270 grams per day without complaining.

Neither our endocrinologist nor Bo-In Lee wanted to talk to one another, but they both agreed that we should maintain at least a one-unit dose of insulin as long as possible to rest Danny's remaining islet cells. The problem was that Danny had several low blood sugar events, even on that small dose, and in the end, everyone decided to end his shots as long as he was carefully monitored.

By mid-April, three months after diagnosis, Danny was off insulin entirely!

We had an indescribable amount of freedom. Danny ran through the neighborhood without supervision, slept over at friends' houses (no one had offered to keep him for that long after his diagnosis), and Brian and I were able to sleep through the night. All I carried with me on short trips with Danny were glucose tabs. We continued with a carefully measured diet, regular blood sugar testing, and fewer carbohydrates when his blood sugar ran high. His blood sugar average for the first two weeks in May was 120. He did have a low of 59 and a high of 325, but his body always returned within range by itself.

This period without insulin gave our family an almost ecstatic sense of freedom, which we didn't know we valued so highly until we regained it. Overall Brian and Danny were even keeled. I still found my tension level rising every time Danny's blood sugar ran high as I wondered if this was the end of his insulin-free period. Thankfully, most of the time he was in range, and I wanted to shout for joy. We were all united in the belief that even if he went back on large doses of insulin for the rest of his life, we were experiencing a genuine miracle.

Our whole family was having a honeymoon.

Positive Changes in Our Family

In May, for the first time, I was able to step back and look at some of the ways we'd changed as a family. It dawned on me that diabetes was like most hardships, bringing blessings along with the challenges. We were eating healthier than we ever had and exercising more, and we were much more grateful for small joys in our everyday life. Danny wasn't the only one reveling in being the center of loving attention. The rest of us found it deeply reassuring to know that we were loved by so many people outside our immediate family. We felt held by a wider community. Also, because we needed to rely upon one another in a way we'd never had to in the past, we'd gotten closer to each other, more trusting and more connected.

During the first months, dinnertime had been tense and disjointed; there were too many food and insulin decisions to make, along with phone calls to doctors and dealing with Danny's complaints. To keep the kids busy, I'd put them in charge of setting the table with colorful place mats while Brian and I huddled over our papers and figured out what to do. Now that Danny was off insulin, we still set a nice table and lingered over dinner, but instead of discussing numbers and needles, we talked about the upcoming soccer season, school, or summer plans.

Danny was an inch taller and years more mature than he'd been four months earlier. He'd learned to listen to his body's messages and to be relatively content with an apple when the kids around him were eating donuts. He still complained about the food, but he took blood tests and went to all his appointments without self-pity. Brian, Jessie, and I had tremendous respect for how he'd handled himself in a variety of difficult situations and accepted having fewer freedoms than his friends did. Remarkably, he'd handled all these life changes without visible resentment or anger. Unless we brought up his diabetes, he rarely mentioned it, and when he did, it was usually to ask a practical question like, "Should I test while I'm at Zach's house?"

Jessie, meanwhile, had matured as well. She'd made it a point to learn everything there was to know about Danny's care, and she was increasingly attuned to his emotional as well as his physical states. Though she often expressed her affection and sympathy for him, she felt free to say she was glad she hadn't been the one to get diabetes. As far as I could tell, she hadn't been sidetracked from her own interests by her brother's illness. In fact, she'd become much more independent, reaching out to friends and family with more energy than ever.

From the beginning, I'd made an effort to spend time alone with Jessie, taking her out to dinner or for a walk around the neighborhood while Brian stayed home with Danny, but I was often distracted. Now that things were easier, her father and I made a point of reading to her at bedtime or helping her with one of the art projects she always had going.

Brian breathed a sigh of relief and went back to his regular work schedule. He returned to jujitsu practice one night a week, and we went out on dates together. The fun and laughter came back.

Because this experience was so precious, I was more committed than ever to prolonging it. Though I hadn't found a word about extending the honeymoon, it seemed to me that since resting allowed the islet cells to produce more insulin, stress might make the islet cells die more quickly. Danny's body could be stressed by too many carbohydrates or not enough exercise, so I tried to prepare more low-carbohydrate foods that he'd be willing to eat; there weren't many. We continued to walk and go for bike rides. Since the doctors had said that the honeymoon was usually brought to an end by a cold or the flu, I tried to keep him away from kids who were sick.

A Typical Day

Four months after his diagnosis, this was a day in Danny's life:

Danny and Brian woke at six o'clock and went downstairs to the kitchen where Danny tested his blood sugar level. It was 103. He had a breakfast smoothie of whole milk and frozen banana, strawberries and blueberries, which contained forty carbohydrates. He then took his Korean herbs, acidophilus, Chlorocaps, evening primrose oil, a multivitamin, and a B-vitamin.

For lunch, Brian packed an organic peanut butter and jelly sandwich on oat bran bread and sliced peppers, carrots and cucumber, which contained forty carbohydrates. He included two snacks in Danny's backpack: a bag of corn puffs and a single serving of applesauce for ten o'clock, which totaled thirty carbohydrates, and a bag of popcorn for two thirty in the afternoon, which had fifteen. At this point, we had reduced his carbohydrate intake from 270 grams per day to approximately 210.

Danny was getting no insulin. At lunch, at his desk in the classroom, he tested his blood sugar and wrote it down on his lunch box label. Three days earlier, he'd been 68 at lunch. He took a glucose tab to raise his number before he ate his meal. Today he was 281, with no discernible difference in our routine. Because he was over 240, he excused himself to go to the bathroom and checked for ketones in his urine. The test strip showed none and he returned to his classroom.

When Danny got home at three thirty in the afternoon, he was 141. For his four o'clock snack, he was very hungry, and I gave him some cut vegetables, slices of apple, a few chunks of cheese, and some peanut butter on celery, which added up to thirty carbohydrates. In response he said, "I'm sick of all that. I'm starving." He tended to feel his food limitations most intensely after school, and he often took out his frustrations on me.

On this day, after he ate his snack, he complained that there was nothing to eat in the house. The kitchen was stocked with things he usually liked and could eat any time. I offered him pepperoni, organic beef hot dogs, sliced chicken, and cheese sticks, but he said he wanted ice cream or Doritos or a soda. When Danny had a friend over or had soccer practice, food wasn't an issue, but today he was miserable.

I handed him some glucose tabs for his pocket and encouraged him to go outside and ride his bike with his friends. He came in at six, and his blood sugar number was 80. For dinner, I served organic steak tips, steamed broccoli, a salad with Danny's favorite ranch dressing, and fruit salad. Even though he ate as much as he wanted, he still complained that he was never going to get enough food.

Brian, who had just arrived home, put his arm around him and said, "Buddy, don't worry. We're going to make sure you're full before this meal is over," while I tried not to growl at him for being ungrateful and whiny. We encouraged him to eat until he was sure he was full. At dinner, he had another round of supplements.

After dinner it was still light outside, so Brian, Danny, and Jessie played basketball with the neighborhood kids while I cleaned up. When they came back in, I tested Danny and gave him blueberries with whipped cream, containing fifteen carbohydrates, for a bedtime snack. He complained with great dramatic flourishes that he was starving again, but Brian and I were firm that it was time for bed and he was asleep within minutes.

I was too tense to sleep myself. Danny's complaints were driving me crazy. I got up and found a recipe for homemade ice cream, sweetened with maple syrup and Stevia, an herbal sweetener that doesn't affect blood sugar levels, and a recipe for nut cookies that had only six carbohydrates each. I was determined to find some nutritious, sweet snacks he could eat. Armed with new recipes to try in the morning, I went to bed.

Going Camping as a Family

When my sister and I were in our early teens, my parents purchased some land in Vermont where we often pitched a tent. After years of rain-soaked adventures, our family built a two-room cabin out of scrap lumber. It wasn't beautiful and had no electricity or running water, but it was dry and we all loved cooking food over the stone-rimmed campfire in our outdoor "kitchen." This year everyone in my family was looking forward to lying in the field on our backs, watching fire-flies and shooting stars.

Brian and I had to admit to each other that we were scared. There was no phone and the nearest hospital was twenty-five minutes away. What if Danny had a hypoglycemic event at night? All we'd have was a flashlight. How would we reach anyone for help? Finally, I came up with an idea. I called the Vermont phone company and discovered there was a telephone pole on the road nearby. For a small fee, they could hook us up. In Vermont, 9-1-1 was free, and within a week, the cabin was connected with the outside world.

We arrived on the land for Memorial Day weekend. The four-hour ride boosted Danny's numbers to 400 on Friday night, but he was up and out in the morning, getting the breakfast fire going before Brian and I woke up. I looked out the screen door at Danny's face. He was deep in concentration, carefully feeding the fire small branches he'd gathered in the woods. He moved with assurance and purpose, looking serene and at ease. His body was stronger and slimmer than ever. You'd never guess that this child was coping with a major illness. Danny, the source of our unceasing worry and broken sleep, was thriving.

I knew in that moment that I wanted to be more like him.

Danny had maintained a sense of quiet confidence. He'd adjusted to the huge changes required of him more easily than I had, allowing new circumstances to make new demands. I think he was content to let us do the fussing and worrying for him. I stood there, feeling proud of him. As Danny put the grate over the fire pit, I resolved to carry my burden more lightly, to accomplish my various jobs without adding unnecessary anxiety, to attend to each task as Danny was attending to the fire, one thing at a time.

I wasn't always able to live up to that resolution, or even to remember that I wanted to, but each time we went camping that summer, I was reminded of the ease that came from doing one task at a time. Agonizing over things didn't make the job easier in any way; at certain blessed times you could simply leave the worry out of it.

The Challenging Role of Caretaker

When Danny was off insulin for three weeks, the relief we felt was indescribable. Without worrying about low blood sugar, comas, or seizures, I felt like we were a normal family for the first time since Danny's diagnosis. To our dismay, however, in mid-May his blood sugar numbers started to rise again. After consulting with our endocrinologist, we started him in the morning on Ultralente, long-acting insulin, with small doses of quick-acting Humalog at meal times. The doctors felt their prediction had been confirmed. They foresaw a steady climb, probably very precipitous, until Danny was back to twenty units of insulin per day.

Our primary goal remained trying to keep Danny's blood sugar level between 80 and 180. We had some days when all his numbers were in range, but there were many more when none of them fell into place. We were hitting about 50 percent. Our doctor felt this was very good. We didn't. I reread *Dr. Bernstein's Diabetes Solution*. He recommended testing before each meal or snack and giving many tiny, carefully calibrated shots of insulin during the day. Our endocrinologist, however, did not suggest this. His stated goal for us was to keep Danny's life as normal as possible and to minimize how much diabetes interfered with his activities.

Brian and I felt caught in an untenable position. Many daily tests and shots gave Danny a greater chance of targeted blood sugars and a healthier future. Giving only two to three shots while letting him eat what the other kids were eating resulted in a more normal, less hassled life. All parents of a child with juvenile diabetes hold in their hands not only their child's day-to-day life, but his or her future health as well. Where is the middle road between making a child feel overwhelmed by his illness on the one hand and risking terrible future consequences on the other?

Some days I could sit back and say that we had no control over the long-term course of Danny's illness. I found comfort in the belief that we were doing the best we could and that we couldn't know what the future would bring. A cure could be found tomorrow. New technology might give him an artificial pancreas. He could be hit by another car. In my philosophical moments, decisions became easier because all I could do was try my best. I'd think, "Danny has his own path, I have mine, and we have to accept whatever life brings us." At those times, I'd feel peaceful and strong.

However, when I had to decide whether to interrupt him for an extra dose of insulin or let him continue playing with a friend, I felt painfully conflicted. One voice would say, "Let him be a kid," and the other would respond, "Every high leaves its mark. Every low is another assault on his system. You're irresponsible if you don't step in." As a result, I was still lying in bed most nights, my head a jumble of thoughts, trying to come up with some plan, some treatment, some diet, to make the next day's numbers improve.

CHAPTER 5

▼

The Second Six Months

Changing Our Diet

At the end of July, Danny was on a minimal dose of Ultralente and a few 0.5 unit shots of Humalog. I was exhilarated that his honeymoon was continuing and remembered that when Danny was first diagnosed, I'd come across a book called *The Raw Family* by Victoria Boutenko at our local health food store. Hers was the only story I'd ever read about a child healing completely from Type 1 diabetes. Rejecting insulin, she'd put her son on a diet of raw fruits, vegetables, nuts, seeds, and soaked grains. After months of adjustment, the family became accustomed to their new diet, and her son's symptoms disappeared. I spoke to a friend who'd met the Boutenko family years later. She said that the boy was the picture of health. Although I could not verify that he had actually had Type 1 diabetes, I took this story to heart.

My friend, Nancy, who swore that eating raw foods was relieving her fibromyalgia, lent me some of her raw food cookbooks: *The Raw Truth: The Art of Loving Foods* by Jeremy A. Safron and Renee Underkoffler and *The Raw Gourmet* by Nomi Shannon. She introduced me to several people on this diet. All of them raved about the health benefits of eating enzyme-rich food that had not been cooked and insisted that they had more energy and zest for life. They reported that their health problems had cleared up and swore they'd never go back to using a stove or microwave again.

I knew I couldn't do this with our family. I couldn't imagine foregoing cookouts, eating at other people's houses or in restaurants, or shopping only in the produce section. The strain would be too much to inflict on all of us—even if there was a chance that Danny's health might improve.

Nevertheless, there was no reason I couldn't make a salad with each meal and serve raw vegetables as often as cooked ones. We were already eating fresh and frozen fruit in smoothies and fruit salad, which provided some enzymes to help with digestion. I decided to introduce bread made from sprouted wheat. I also started soaking raw nuts and cooking them at low temperatures, which protected their enzymes. I substituted them for the roasted ones Danny was eating in large quantities.

Brian agreed that the inclusion of enzyme-rich raw food could be a good move for the whole family. We also reconsidered Bo-In Lee's suggestion to take Danny off wheat and dairy. We all had frequent colds and fevers, Jessie and Brian had eczema, and Danny still had occasional rashes. Perhaps these things were related to food allergies.

The problem was finding a way to eat differently without driving everyone crazy. I didn't want to end up being a traffic cop stationed in front of the fridge. I decided the ideal time to begin would be during our vacation in August. We'd give up wheat, dairy, sugar, and processed foods. I'd bring along bags of supplies from our health food store. I could buy freshly picked fruits and vegetables from a local farm stand and meat and seafood from local stores. No one would feel deprived.

That first morning I baked peach crumble for breakfast. The recipe called for rolled oats that had been soaked overnight, fresh peaches, frozen berries, and butter. We sweetened our coffee and tea with a sweet herb called Stevia, which is widely available in supermarkets, and drank soy and almond milk instead of cow's milk. For lunch, we put raw almond butter and organic peanut butter on rice cakes and learned how to make our own salad dressings. We made ice cream from blended frozen fruit for dessert. At dinner, we had ribs on the grill, corn on the cob, and another salad. I'd been told you could eat corn raw so I didn't boil it. We each tentatively took a bite and were amazed at how sweet and fresh it tasted. After that, we didn't cook it. I prepared a pie for dessert, making the crust from almonds and cashews and the filling by blending bananas, strawberries, blueberries, and unsweetened cocoa. Everyone loved it.

Luckily, the kids took our new way of eating as a family challenge and helped with the planning and cooking. Brian and I agreed we'd never felt better. We both had more energy, needed less sleep, and never felt hungry. The kids reported feeling no difference, but this was the first vacation we'd taken during which no one gained weight. In addition, we exercised every day. The whole family took long bike rides, Danny's personal best being fourteen miles one day while Jessie covered ten.

To our delight, Danny's numbers began steadily dropping and by the end of vacation, he was off insulin again!

We had several scares when his numbers dropped too low without any insulin at all. At one point, we called the hospital to consult the endocrinologist-on-call, and he said it could be the result of his pancreas giving out too much insulin before quitting completely. Predictably, he urged us to prepare ourselves for the end of the honeymoon. I didn't bother to ask whether we were eating so well that Danny's pancreas was having a party.

"Food is one of those subjects where we've changed for the better and I wouldn't go back," Jessie said one evening at dinner. "This vacation's been hard because we couldn't have ice cream every day the way we used to. I'm glad you made the ice cream cake thing with the nuts for crust and smoothies in layers because that was really good."

I asked her how she'd describe the way we eat now.

"I like that our whole family eats the same food as Danny," she said. "It's a healthy way to eat. I used to eat sweets a lot, but I'm not a big dessert person anymore. It's still hard to have to eat at the same time every night and have a salad with every meal, plus, we have a lot of meat, which I don't really like, but I'm glad you looked into nutrition. I'm pretty much used to oatmeal bread, and I know white flour isn't good for you. I like using Stevia instead of sugar, but it doesn't taste the same.

"When I'm home, I eat what everyone else does because there's nothing else around. You don't buy anything with sugar or white flour, like store-bought cookies. I don't really mind the changes, except when you expect us to eat potato chips that don't taste good." She grinned. "I'm 'specially glad that when I'm out of the house, I can eat whatever I want."

Before we returned home from vacation, I called my mother and asked her to get rid of everything in our house containing wheat, dairy, and sugar. We were convinced that diet was one of the reasons that Danny was off insulin again, and for a while, we continued avoiding these things. However, what had seemed normal while we were away was really a burden when we got home. Back home, we gave in to the temptations of wedding food, birthday treats, restaurants, and meals at friends' houses. Yet, our diet was still better than it had been, and everyone was feeling healthier.

Providing meals was still far from easy. Danny, in particular, continued to be an incredibly fussy eater and, although we made him taste everything, he refused to eat anything that didn't appeal to him right that moment. We'd always said, "Taste everything. If you don't like it, you can have a bowl of cereal," but we couldn't do that now because a bowl of cereal contained sixty-five carbohydrates and wouldn't fill him. I desperately wanted a dinner that wasn't spoiled by a struggle over food.

One night I served pork chops with pineapple, a big salad, roasted asparagus, and leftover vegetable chowder. I sat down to dinner feeling relaxed and confident because Danny had eaten this in the past. He took one look at his dish and said, "Can I have something else?"

In an instant, I was angry and frustrated. I refused to answer, and Jessie ended up browbeating Danny into silence. In the end, he ate the salad and the tips of the asparagus while Jessie commented that although the pork looked disgusting, she'd eat the other stuff. I ended up giving them a tight-lipped lecture about how there were starving kids who'd give anything for this meal. At this point in our life, I dreaded dinnertime and daydreamed about having a cook.

The Roller Coaster Ride: On Insulin Again

By the end of the summer, I'd gotten lax about our diet. We were also getting less daily exercise. Danny's numbers started to rise, and he needed long-acting insulin again. This time the doctors prescribed Lantus, a new 18-to 24-hour insulin that was less likely to cause low blood sugars. Brian and I began checking Danny in the middle of the night again. Although we didn't set up the baby monitor, we slept lightly. I wanted to go back to our vacation diet, but no one else did and I was too discouraged to argue. I was so busy trying to keep up with daily demands that I couldn't rally to make any more changes.

It didn't help that our friends and family assumed that after eight months, we were now out of crisis. Most people believe that diabetes is a disease you get under control, and then you move on. We'd thought that ourselves. Since Danny looked and acted normal, friends and acquaintances expected us to return to our former lives and pick up where we'd left off. Meals no longer came from the Caring Committee at church, people no longer called to ask what they could do, and if someone wondered how Danny was, they expected a simple "fine" in reply. I didn't want to continue burdening others with my worries and needs. It seemed time to keep them to myself.

After all, we were bike-riding all over town, going to the beach, and hanging out with friends. It certainly looked to the outside world that we were over the worst of it, and we were. Yet at home, on the chart where we carefully recorded every one of Danny's numbers and meals, we were still riding an unpredictable roller coaster.

In September, nine months after his diagnosis, Danny's Hemoglobin A1c number was 7.8. Our endocrinology team was pleased, but we were aware that in spite of all our efforts, Danny's numbers had barely improved. I had heard that extreme highs and lows could average out to look deceptively good on this test. I thought the number was too high, but wasn't confident enough to say so. I'd been told that blood sugar levels are easier to control during the honeymoon. Where would his numbers be when his insulin needs rose? Meanwhile Danny remained blissfully unaware of any of the future consequences of juvenile diabetes. He just knew that we were trying to keep him between 80 and 180 in order to keep him from feeling sick, and he was fine with that.

Coping with a Fever

In early September, my sister Julie had her second child, a boy named Luke. I'd just returned from visiting them in the hospital when Danny came home from school with a fever of 101 degrees. I went on high alert. I didn't want us back in the hospital. He'd had a half unit of long-acting Lantus that morning and lows all day. At lunch, he'd been 72. Now, feverish, he lay on the couch all afternoon. No exercise and a fever meant higher numbers. Asleep at ten thirty that night, he was 313. Brian and I decided not to give him more insulin because we were afraid that his blood sugar would drop when his fever broke.

Danny woke up the next morning with a blood sugar of 181. We gave him his regular 0.5 of Humalog and 0.5 of Lantus and kept him home from school, resting. His numbers kept rising. By ten o'clock that morning, he was 244. After two-thirds of a unit of Humalog, at lunch he was 155, so I gave him another 0.5 of Humalog. He complained about so many shots.

During the day, the coordinator of a well-respected diabetes research center in Colorado returned my call. I gave her a quick overview of Danny's honeymoon and asked whether her center was looking into prolonging honeymoons or complementary treatments. She paused, and then said firmly, "I want you to know that in all our experience at the center with parents who think they're making a difference by trying alternative treatments, in one hundred percent of the cases it ultimately makes no difference. Parents spend time, energy, and money, but the honeymoon always ends."

She said that in every case the child had gotten a virus that elevated the blood sugar, which then never came down. I thanked her for her time and got off the phone, feeling sick myself. Maybe this virus was the one that would put Danny on twenty units forever. Worse was the feeling that maybe we were fooling ourselves. All our unconventional attempts to help Danny probably looked ridiculous to his doctors.

By that afternoon, Danny was feeling better and his fever was down. Aside from a cough, he seemed healthy. In spite of my discouragement, I decided to keep his acupuncture appointment. Danny tested himself in the car. At four o'clock, before his snack, he was 380. I gave him one unit of Humalog.

During the treatment, Bo-In Lee pulled me aside and told me he thought the virus was attacking Danny's pancreas. Everyone said that things were going to be worse after the honeymoon was over. I kept repeating, *I can only do what I can do,* but it didn't help. I was a mother, and my son's body was under attack. I felt a rising panic.

I steeled myself because Danny needed a meal. We went to our favorite Thai restaurant before heading home. When I tested him before the meal, he was 389. I prepared a unit and a half of Humalog. He looked up at me with his big brown eyes and said, "Please, Mom, no more shots."

Blinking back tears, I gave Danny the shot anyway. It was dangerous for him to have high blood sugars for too long. I tried to stay as calm as possible, but I couldn't seem to swallow, and I felt scared being alone with him so far from home. I asked him to urinate on a ketone test strip, and I felt reassured when it came back negative. I took him home and put him to bed. At ten fifteen, he was 288 in his sleep. In one day, I'd given my son six shots, and I hadn't once gotten his blood sugar numbers within an acceptable range.

That night in bed, filled with doubts, I turned to Brian. "How do we know we're doing the right thing?" I asked. "Should we stop the acupuncture? Should I have given him even more insulin? Am I putting all this energy into changing our diet for nothing?"

All Brian said was, "Hon, we're doing the best we can."

For some reason, it was the perfect thing to say. He was right. All we could do was keep putting one foot in front of the other. Just like ants who can't see the big picture, but continue to do their one specialized job, you do what you have to do and trust that there's some reason for it.

The next day Danny woke up at 161 and was in the 200s all day. He got five shots, but didn't complain.

I didn't want to increase Danny's insulin too quickly because two days ago, these same amounts of insulin would have sent his blood sugar levels dropping through the floor. I stood by helplessly as his numbers remained high. I kept trying to surrender to the flow of events, to accept that his numbers were beyond my control. I kept saying to myself, "This is his life. I'm just here to help as best I can."

Thursday morning, Danny woke up with a blood sugar of 130. I sent him off to school with my fingers crossed, and despite my nervousness, he finished the day with four shots and only one number over 200. We thought of giving him another shot at dinner, but he said he'd rather go without carbohydrates, so he ate a salad with ranch dressing and asparagus. He had a big helping of blueberries with whipped cream for his bedtime snack. At ten thirty, asleep, he was 172.

Roland came at four thirty the next day to do his healing work. He listened to my story about the woman at the research center and reminded me that we hadn't changed our eating habits, increased Danny's exercise, or tried acupuncture solely for his pancreas. Our one true goal was to help him be as healthy and happy as possible and simply giving him insulin wasn't going to accomplish that. "Laura," Roland said, "as long as we seem to be making the quality of Danny's life better, we're going to keep going."

Roland's certainty made me aware of how confused I was. I felt as if someone had smashed the compass that was guiding me through uncharted territory. He reminded me once again of the importance of unbroken sleep and having people with whom you can think aloud. Sometimes I lost my perspective just because I was so tired and I needed someone else's spirit to recharge mine.

Changing to Another Diabetes Team

During our first six months, we were grateful to our endocrinologist and our nurse diabetes educator for their warmth and caring. Our doctor had an appointment at a prestigious medical school and was at the top of his field. He looked Danny straight in the eye and asked him how he was, what sports he played, and how he felt about his diabetes. They both helped us regulate his blood sugars to the best of their ability and reassured us when we were scared. We saw one of them every three months and called our nurse whenever we needed advice.

By October, ten months later, we were unhappy. Actually, I was unhappy and after a while, Brian agreed to look elsewhere. I had so many unanswered questions about the glycemic index and about the effect of whole foods versus processed ones. I wondered if other families had tried acupuncture or vitamin supplements. Was it true that giving your child fewer carbohydrates, and therefore less insulin, put less stress on his system? Ultimately, we wanted a medical team that was open-minded and could talk to us about these issues.

Recently, I had e-mailed a well-respected diabetes researcher in the Midwest about the course of Danny's disease. He'd acknowledged that Danny's situation was unusual, although not unheard of, and suggested we test him for antibodies to be certain that he didn't have Type 2 diabetes instead. I forwarded the e-mail to our nurse diabetes educator, and at our next appointment, Danny had this test along with his Hemoglobin A1c.

I was focused on Danny's now seven-month honeymoon, and this was clearly making our doctor nervous. He never missed an opportunity to warn about the dangers of "false hope," two words I don't think should ever go together. He said that inevitably Danny's insulin needs would end up as high as everyone else's was, and that therefore we shouldn't make the honeymoon an issue. When we mentioned diet or acupuncture, he expressed no interest except to urge us to "do no harm." I realized before Brian did that if we wanted a truly open and trusting relationship with our medical team, we had to find a better match.

All summer I'd looked for another endocrinology team. I used words like "holistic," "whole foods nutrition," and "alternative," searching for someone who was curious, excited about his or her work, and eager to learn more. All the doctors and nurses I knew shook their heads. Finally, my mother-in-law, Anne, suggested I get in touch with the head of the department of Eastern and Western medicine at a university nearby, and he suggested that we contact an endocrinologist named Dr. M. He described her as very open-minded and thought she'd be a wonderful doctor for our family. When I called, however, her practice was full so the receptionist gave us an appointment with her colleague, Dr. J, for early December.

An Unexplainable Crisis

After Danny had the flu, it took a couple of weeks of acupuncture and weekly visits from Roland to get Danny back down to one unit of Lantus again. Even on days without exercise, his pancreas kept him in remarkably good control. We had a few particularly stable days in late October, and Brian and I relaxed. It seemed like we were finally getting the hang of keeping Danny's blood sugar levels in goal range.

The next Saturday Danny woke up at 131. Throughout the day, his numbers were just a little higher than usual. As we sat down to dinner at a restaurant that evening, Danny was 305. We gave him one unit of Humalog and proceeded to enjoy our meal. Danny was asleep by eight thirty.

At eleven, Brian went in to check Danny's blood sugar. His reading was off the meter, which only goes to 500. Beyond that, it just reads "high." This had never happened before, and we were both very frightened. We reached the endocrinologist on call, and he said there was no formula for treating children on so little insulin. He suggested giving Danny one more unit of Humalog and testing him again in an hour. We could tell that he was taking a wild guess. His advice didn't reassure us.

The idea of giving Danny a shot in his belly while he was sleeping was so unnerving that I asked Brian to do it. I hovered in the hallway and listened to Danny's little voice go, "Ow! Ow!" Then I helped him into the bathroom where he urinated on a test strip. The strip turned tan, which meant no ketones.

We set our alarm for 12:30 AM. Brian slept and I lay awake for an hour and a half, my eyes fixed on the ceiling, alert for any signs of distress. At 12:36 AM, Danny was 354. No ketones again. Brian set the alarm for 1:30 AM. He slept and I lay awake some more, listening. At 1:42 AM, Danny was 469 so we called the hospital again. The doctor said it was highly unusual for a child's blood sugar to go back up without his having had any food. Predictably, he said, "This is probably the end of the honeymoon."

In the middle of the night, bleary-eyed and half-asleep, Brian and I both confronted the possibility that Danny's diabetes had suddenly taken a turn for the worse.

We tested Danny for ketones again, gave him two-thirds of a unit of Humalog, and set the alarm for 3:15 AM. I may have slept, but if I did, I dreamed I was awake. Brian had a nightmare and woke up sweating. At 3:21 AM, Danny was 289, and we decided it was safe to sleep through the rest of the night.

At breakfast, Danny was 190. Although we were exhausted, we went on a family hike. Danny was outside and moving for five hours straight. We gave Danny four and one-third units of insulin in five separate shots, trying to keep his numbers down. Even then, at our last check of the day, he was 235.

The next morning, to our relief, he woke up at 106. That day, we gave him three units of insulin in three shots. The next day he had two and one-half units of insulin in three shots before seeing Bo-In Lee that afternoon. The next day he was down to two units of insulin and after that, he leveled out at one and one-half units a day with very solid numbers.

No one's ever had any explanation for what happened.

We'd weathered another crisis, and this time we could see a pattern. Every time something unusual happened, we were told authoritatively, without our asking, that Danny's honeymoon was about to end. Finally, it dawned on us that these highly-educated endocrinologists couldn't read Danny's future any better than we could. I vowed not to take doctors' warnings so seriously in the future.

Parties and Halloween

The first year with a child with diabetes calls for many new responses to familiar situations. Holidays and parties suddenly became much more challenging. Believe me, everything is easier the second time around.

Birthday parties were full of temptation, and I had learned to send Danny a low carb snack to eat so that he'd feel full enough to settle for small portions of pizza, cake, and ice cream. With Lantus, which gave him flexibility, he felt secure about making his own decisions and often ate some of the dessert, giving himself extra insulin to cover it. Even though he couldn't eat as much as the other kids could, he was very matter-of-fact, and I had to remind myself not to feel worse about it than he did.

One celebration came unexpectedly. The driver of Danny's school bus spontaneously decided to take all the kids to Dunkin' Donuts after school. Danny arrived home, talking excitedly about which kind of donut each of his friends had chosen. I tried to be lighthearted as I asked, "Well, what did you have?" and he said, quite happily, "I couldn't have a donut with all those carbs. I had my apple." I'd been ready to feel sorry for him, but he didn't feel sorry for himself. He quickly changed the subject to buying new sneakers.

Going to events with other families took a big adjustment. We found that when we relaxed and hung out with our adult friends, we lost track of what Danny was eating. When we got home, his blood sugars would be very high, and we'd have to get up at all hours of the night to give him shots of insulin, shaking our heads about how stupid we'd been. We finally learned that we had to stay alert because our lapses always ended up at Danny's expense. It was definitely easier when we ate at home. We tended to make only brief appearances at large get-togethers for that reason.

Now I was especially wary as our first Halloween approached. Jessie suggested we go around the neighborhood, handing out small gifts for people to put into Danny's Halloween bag. She and I had fun at the drugstore, stocking up on such items as a yo-yo, a glow stick, a Matchbox car, and colored pencils. Thankfully, our neighbors loved the idea. Some of them insisted on getting Danny their own special treats. Everyone seemed happy to cooperate.

We asked Danny what he wanted to do with the candy he got trick-or-treating. First, he considered giving it to the homeless shelter, but on second thought, he was more excited about selling it to his father who'd offered him ten cents apiece. In the end, Halloween turned out to be a great success. Danny found Halloween as exciting as ever and at the end of the night, he had many things to keep. As the kids sat around our neighborhood bonfire, waiting for the storytelling to begin, Danny's friends were inspecting the surprising items in his bag and seemed to be looking at his diabetes in a new light.

At one point Danny came over and told Brian he needed a shot because he'd eaten two pieces of candy. We were relieved that he hadn't hidden it from us. At bedtime, and in the middle of the night, Danny's numbers were fine. We'd survived our first Halloween.

Working on My Attitude

Two months before our one-year mark, we hit the lowest point in our journey emotionally. At the beginning of November, test results revealed Danny's antibodies were alive and active. Now we knew for sure that he was definitely Type 1.

At that same time, Danny's numbers slowly began to climb. Up to now, an evening reading of 300 would have ended up between 100 and 130 in the morning without treatment. Now, with a nighttime number half that amount, it took a shot of insulin to bring his morning blood sugar into that range.

Danny was declaring he hated food that he'd been happy to eat just days before, and even bursting into tears at the table. I found myself wanting to say, "Eat what we put in front of you or go to bed hungry," but his illness meant that I had to keep trying to please him. These daily ricochets between flashes of anger and moments of remorse were tying my stomach into knots.

Our family was getting up at six o'clock in the morning to get through the whole diabetes routine. By afternoon, I was tired. I was forgetting things and letting others slide, only to be reminded by Danny's numbers that he was the one who suffered. Roland had stopped coming because he no longer worked nearby, and I realized how much his presence had kept me motivated and on track. I needed to be vigilant at all times because I didn't have a duplicate to relieve me, and in spite of the support of my husband and family, I still felt like I was only staying afloat by ceaselessly treading water. Whenever I had a quiet moment to myself, I noticed how exhausted I was, mentally as much as physically.

One of the things that kept me going during this period was my faith. Brian and I believed that the four of us chose each other on a very deep level. We were meant to be together. To us this meant that our child had diabetes for a reason, even though we didn't know what it was. We also had faith that the challenges we faced could make us stronger because we'd been through so much before this. When I was scared or tired, I tended to lose my focus, but eventually I would hear a small still voice saying that there was a greater purpose for all of us, and my energy and confidence would return.

Brian and I have never been people who took things lying down. It was clear that Danny's diabetes was now a given in our lives, but we refused to give up trying to affect the outcome. We were intrigued by a book called *The Law and the Promise* by a man named Neville who believed that human thought could shape reality. He suggested taking several minutes to put yourself, in your mind's eye, into a future moment when your wishes had been fulfilled and to imagine how wonderful you'd feel. We experienced this practice of visualization as a blessing because it enabled us to infuse ourselves with positive feelings and to escape, if only for a short while, being worn down and worn out by feelings of helplessness and exhaustion.

Sometimes when Danny's numbers were high, we'd lie in bed together and imagine ourselves the following night, remarking on how low and predictable Danny's numbers had been. During those few minutes, we could feel ourselves relaxing as we imagined the relief of a day with Danny's numbers in the 80s and 90s.

We did it for our own sakes, but sometimes we had results. During our August vacation, we repeatedly imagined how wonderful it was going to feel to have Danny tell our medical team that he was off insulin. We went through that process every night for a week while Danny's need for insulin slowly and steadily kept dropping. We weren't sure our prayer had made a difference, but it was an awe-inspiring experience for us when Danny actually walked into the nurse's office and made his declaration.

Despite our distress, Brian and I used this same technique the night Danny registered off the meter. We imagined the relief and gratitude we'd feel when Danny's numbers went back down again and eventually, what we imagined became reality. I truly believe that being able to access positive feelings when things looked bleak was part of the reason Danny was functioning so well. Whether or not we created any physical changes, allowing reassuring images to renew our energy and enthusiasm was a far better way to spend our sleepless nights than worrying.

Danny's Weeklong School Trip

Late in November, I spent a week accompanying Danny and his third grade class to the Hawthorne Valley Farm Camp in Ghent, New York. Danny hiked up a mountain, mucked out the cow barn, and played football with his friends. He rode a horse, made apple cider, chopped and stacked wood, and was outdoors from morning to night, even in the rain. He ate only biodynamic, organic vegetarian food. On Monday when we arrived, he was on 1.5 units of long-acting insulin a day. Even with extra carbohydrates, like maple syrup, honey, whole grain pancakes, and raisins, he still had lows every day and by Friday, he was having significant lows on one unit of Lantus. All week, he never went over 193.

I had fun. The kids and the chaperones all played and explored the farm as a group. Diabetes was a small and insignificant part of my days with Danny. I gave him his shot each morning, and every time he tested, there was nothing to figure out and nothing to do except tell him to enjoy himself. Meals were provided, and exercise was built in. It was heavenly.

On Thursday, Danny heard that the farm had an overnight summer camp and was sure he wanted to come back. "Two weeks, Mom," he said. "I can't wait." That night, I sidled up to Gisela, the camp's nurse, prepared for the possibility of rejection, or worse, disbelief. Instead, she told me that although she'd never taken care of a child with diabetes before, she'd like to make it possible. We agreed to talk in the spring and decide whether it was too much for her or not. She was warm and caring, the kind of person I felt I could trust, and Danny had a hungry look in his eye when he asked if he could come back. I hoped we could work it out.

As soon as we returned home, Danny's need for insulin began to climb.

On the farm, his average wake-up number was 110. Back home he averaged around 140. He went to school each day, had a half hour of recess twice a day, then came home and complained that he was tired, it was freezing outside, and he didn't want to exercise. Sometimes I managed to get him down to the basement to do twenty minutes on a stationery bike, wrestle with me, or take a half-hour walk, but his exercise was limited and his numbers were unpredictable.

On the farm, he only got one shot a day. Now he was getting two or three. We were both shocked to see the difference in his blood sugars immediately after his return. I asked Danny how he felt everything was going. "Not good," he said. He didn't want to increase his insulin because the more insulin in a shot, the more it hurt him. He didn't want to see more of Bo-In Lee because of the drive, and he didn't want to eat the type of food they served at the farm.

For the millionth time, I wished I had someone who understood which factor had made the difference. More than a cook, more than a duplicate, more than anything, I wanted someone to tell me what to do.

Meeting Our New Diabetes Team

On a Thursday in early December, I took Jessie and Danny out of school early and met Brian at the new hospital for our first appointment with Dr. J. We were excited and optimistic. Even though the doctor walked into the examining room thirty minutes late, we were still all beaming at her. Surprisingly, she barely looked at us. She seemed more competent and well-versed in the latest research than our team at the last hospital; she did a thorough and professional physical exam on Danny in the hour we spent together. However, she knew nothing about acupuncture, and she expressed no interest in our experience with alternative treatments. She said to talk about diet with the nutritionist.

When she looked at the records we'd kept so conscientiously and made no comment on how much care had gone into their keeping, I started to feel discouraged.

"Is this type of record keeping par for the course?" I asked, hoping for just a little pat on the head. "Yes," she replied.

Dr. J also informed us that her son had had a two-year honeymoon. She told us that the average honeymoon was six to nine months and that Danny was well within the norm, in contrast to my findings that the average honeymoon was more likely to run from several weeks to several months.

I felt more and more disappointed as the appointment progressed. I also found myself resisting her insistence that no matter what we did, it wouldn't affect the outcome of Danny's disease. At one point, I got teary, and then I realized I couldn't possibly cry in front of a doctor who wouldn't meet my eyes. When Dr. J left the room so that Danny could change, Jessie said to me with a stricken look, "You can't possibly make Danny have her as a doctor."

At the end of the hour, Dr. J sent us off to the diabetes nurse educator. She'd been incredibly impersonal. I'd assumed that we'd been brought together because she was meant to be our doctor. Now, even though Jessie had been turned off and Brian had already rolled his eyes at me, I didn't know what to think.

We saw our new nurse diabetes educator for an hour. She was much more personable and communicative. When we expressed our frustration at Danny's inconsistent numbers, she was reassuring. She explained that it's easier for an adult to keep his numbers within a certain range because each day he can go to work at the same time, eat the same lunch, and exercise regularly. Children are much harder to regulate or predict because they have gym on Tuesday and soccer practice that gets rained out on Friday. I felt good about the relationship, but she asked no questions about alternative treatments or our changing diet when we mentioned them.

When the nurse saw Danny's numbers, she said we were in the good-to-excellent range in terms of managing his blood sugar, and although there might be an illusion of control with diabetes, she impressed upon us that we could never expect ourselves to do better than we were doing. She said that if we had reasonable expectations, we'd have a much easier time of it in the long haul. A year later, we would find that we could do much better, but at the time, we believed her. Our family consensus was that we liked her a lot.

Our third hour-long appointment was with the nutritionist. She put Danny's current diet into her computer and found it was meeting all his nutritional needs. She felt that his carbohydrate intake was a bit low, but didn't suggest we change anything. When we started to explain why we ate a whole foods diet and avoided artificial ingredients, she quickly responded that, "every family has to do what it has to do."

As we talked further, it became clear that she didn't value natural sweeteners over artificial or whole-wheat flour over white, even though a study in the *American Journal of Clinical Nutrition* had shown that higher whole grain intake is associated with increased sensitivity to the action of insulin. She explained her philosophy by saying, "You tailor the diet to what the child will eat."

I wish I'd said that rather than tailoring the diet to what the child will eat, she'd do better encouraging parents to improve the whole family's diet. I wanted to insist that families without the resources and time I had at my disposal needed handouts on the benefits of healthy eating and suggestions for economically feasible ways to change the foods they ate. I wanted to argue that kids with diabetes, whose organ systems are under stress, need nutrients, natural ingredients, and fewer empty carbohydrates, not further indulgence in the junk food and sweets advertised on television.

I didn't say a word.

I couldn't, with a little voice in my head whispering, "What's wrong with you? Why do you have to question everything? Why can't you let your kid eat whatever he wants and stop fighting him? Maybe she's right and you're just making life hard for yourself."

I desperately wished this medical team had been kindred spirits who'd said, "Wow, you guys are doing a great job. I think all your efforts will truly make a difference in Danny's life." I'd wanted them to care about the things we were trying to do. I'd hoped for some encouragement, but it seemed we weren't any closer to finding what we were looking for.

When we got home, Brian and I looked at the pros and cons: Our first endocrinologist made eye contact, touched Danny, and talked directly to him about his illness. Danny was going to need a doctor like him to relate to when he had his own teenage questions. Yet we had no contact with him beyond one visit every six months, and he'd once joked that with all the reading I was doing, I knew more about current research than he did. At our new hospital, they were clearly briefed on all the latest findings, and there were support groups for all ages in case any of us needed one. We didn't know what to do and since our next appointment was three months away, we decided to pour all our energies into throwing a more-festive-than-ever holiday party and worry about it later.

Family Meetings

Right before Christmas, Brian, my mom, my dad, and I had a two-hour meeting to talk about Danny's progress. I found it extremely helpful because Brian and I were able to talk about the impact these high sugars were having on his body and our fears about Danny's future. My parents mostly listened, so they got a chance to understand where we were and what we'd been going through.

We weren't sure where we should go from here. Was it time to accept that Danny's honeymoon was ending? We decided to take Danny to Bo-In Lee a few times in a row during the vacation week and to ask Roland to see him again. If these things didn't make a difference, it was time to let them go. The meeting filled me with renewed energy. I felt lucky to have my parents as a sounding board, but if I hadn't, I really think parents would be wise to meet every once in a while with caring friends or another family whose child has diabetes. A sympathetic listener can really provide support.

The next day I scheduled three acupuncture treatments and one session with Roland during the holiday break. Danny protested that he didn't want to be so busy, and I promised that even if the treatments worked, he wouldn't have that kind of schedule in the future. In true Danny style, he shrugged and said okay. Because he got nervous before the acupuncture appointments, I promised that we'd go to the toy store, the zoo, or out to dinner afterwards. I loved these adventures because Danny was funny and sweet, but he made sure to remind me that even if he was having fun, this whole arrangement was temporary.

Afterward, it seemed clear that the treatments did help. Instead of continuing to climb, Danny's insulin needs decreased. He'd been starting the day with three units of Lantus and despite several small shots of Humalog during the day, his numbers remained high. Now he was down to 2.5 units of Lantus and 0.5 units of Humalog, and his blood sugar levels were much more reliable. I started to notice little wisps of hope drifting back into my mind and before I went to bed, I started envisioning that Danny was down to two units of insulin in the morning.

Helping Siblings Thrive

In our family, Danny became the center of attention for a very long time. No matter how much effort we made, his care became a constant preoccupation, and Jessie couldn't help but notice that she was getting less attention than she used to. My mother felt that Jessie needed somewhere else to shine, and she explained it to me. "Kids who have a sibling with a chronic illness need sustained contact with caring adults who understand their situation, so that there's a kind of compensation that takes place. Success and encouragement away from home become a way of maintaining their self-esteem, in sports, at school, as a musician or an artist, or in organizations like Girl Scouts, which are devoted to nurturing children."

In our case, Jessie began to work as a babysitter in our Sunday school, and she and one adult were put in charge of the nursery. She took her responsibilities seriously and made a small salary, of which she was very proud. Most important was that our director of religious education trusted and counted on her.

As a result, Jessie was asked to lead the responsive reading from the pulpit on Christmas Eve. She stood there with the church full to overflowing and surveyed the congregation calmly before starting to read slowly and with feeling. Not only was her whole extended family there, but also she was surrounded by caring adults marveling at her poise.

When she joined us, her smile curved all the way up until it was shining in her eyes. I would say she was as happy as any child could be. That's when I realized how important it had been for her to find a niche outside the family. She had found a place of her own where her brother's diabetes had no impact at all.

PART II

▼

The Second Year

CHAPTER 6

▼

The First Six Months

Our One-Year Anniversary

On his actual anniversary, Danny came home from school in an unusually talkative mood. As if we were in the middle of a conversation, he began, "Diabetes is hard. When there's all this food, desserts, and stuff, I can't have it and the other kids do. Sometimes I can have some, but I can only have a small amount of it. It's pretty hard."

I wanted to hear more, so I asked what else was hard to deal with.

"When my blood sugar is low, it's hard to explain, but I feel really tired and not good. I feel really bad. If I feel low during the day, I can test and have some food or tabs, but if I'm really low, I could faint. When I'm high, I feel really tired or really hyper. It depends. Sometimes that means a whole extra shot."

I asked him what had gotten easier.

"I can give myself shots in the stomach or on my arms now. It feels about the same in both places. I don't really mind, but it gets annoying after a while, checking my blood sugar and getting shots all the time. I like having the arm pricker so I don't always have to test my finger. You press a button and it springs into you, and it doesn't really hurt. I know you test me when I'm sleeping because when I wake up in the morning, sometimes I remember you woke me up. It doesn't bother me. I go back to sleep right away. I'm glad I don't have to pay too much attention to the numbers or the blood sugar log. I let you do that."

Danny's morning blood sugars, which started going up again at the one-year mark, indicated there were fewer islet cells left in his pancreas. Now he needed between three and five units of insulin per day, and we had to accept that his pancreatic functioning was definitely diminishing. His honeymoon was on the wane. Brian and I had no idea what other families did to mark the one-year anniversary, but we'd heard that it was a big event psychologically. Celebrating seemed too strange, and ignoring it seemed like a mistake. We decided we'd just talk about the past year at dinner.

First, we said grace, which is the time before meals when each of us mentions something we're grateful for. Danny said, "I'm grateful for this good food and I hope my diabetes goes well next year."

That raised the topic.

I brought up the fact that Danny needed more shots again and that we'd had many changes in one year. Jessie was very open about her disappointment that her brother was back on insulin and her worries about his future. We talked about how quickly technology was advancing, how many researchers had dedicated themselves to finding a cure, and about our confidence that we could manage, no matter how high Danny's insulin needs went. Brian brought up the fact that Danny could practically manage his diabetes on his own. He was giving himself his own shots and helping us decide on the right doses. He seemed to know when he was low and was able to warn us before he was in danger. We concluded that his disease was getting easier to handle every day. Everyone cleared their dishes with smiles on their faces.

For my part, I surprised myself. I seemed to have caught my breath and felt much better than I had in November. I'd actually enjoyed the holidays and the preparations. Danny had finally given up resisting the food I put in front of him, and I loved my time with both kids now that we weren't in constant crisis. Blood sugar tests had become a routine, and Danny's numbers didn't carry the same weight they once had; I was getting used to the ups and downs. For days at a time, I actually felt happy. When I started to think about the future, I reminded myself that there were people with diabetes who avoided long-term consequences and with any luck, Danny would be one of them. Then I crossed my fingers that there would be a cure before Danny had to deal with any of that.

That night I lay in bed with Jessie for a few minutes, and we talked about the changes our family had gone through in the past year, the good and the bad. Jessie started to cry. "I had so much hope. It felt like Danny might go off insulin forever, but he didn't."

My eyes filled with tears and I had to admit, "Me too."

Then the moment passed, and we were both okay again. I realized that even though we'd all been intensely hopeful for a while, disappointment wasn't that crushing. It was nothing we couldn't handle. In fact, looking back, I'm grateful for the time we spent being hopeful. I don't regret it myself or for Jessie and Danny, who seemed to be more resilient than ever. It gave us all time to come to terms with the reality of Danny's illness.

As far as Brian was concerned, Danny's illness hadn't changed the essential nature of our family this year, except perhaps to strengthen it. Most kids become more independent as they get older, but the combination of Danny's attending school out of town and having only a few friends in the neighborhood meant he was actually more available to play with his father than he would have been otherwise.

Brian was also spending more time with Jessie because Danny got so much attention. Before bed, he read to her for half an hour after he read to Danny. She chose the books. They had just finished *The Golden Compass* by Philip Pullman and were about to start the sequel, which he'd bought Jessie for Christmas. Brian had recently taken Jessie shopping for school clothes. Sometimes they watched videos together. Every Friday, Brian had breakfast with one of the kids while their grandfather took the other to breakfast at another restaurant. He also coached Jessie and Danny's soccer teams. In the spring and fall, he left work early for afternoon practices twice a week.

Before Danny was diagnosed, Brian and I sometimes went out together at night. At this point we tried to focus on just being home as a family. In November, we tried to leave both kids overnight with our babysitter Genevieve, but we had to come home after dinner because Danny developed a fever and she got scared. When we left the kids with my parents, Danny ended up having sky-high blood sugars for the next few days. Jessie understood Danny better than anyone else did, so when Brian and I needed time to talk, we took walks in our neighborhood or visited with friends who lived close by. We found that the simpler we made our life, the easier it was to manage.

Danny and my father continued their pattern of going off to the diner for breakfast every other Friday before school. In the beginning Danny went into the bathroom to give himself his insulin shot. At year's end, he just pulled up his shirt at the table and gave himself the shot in the stomach, as if it were nothing special.

One morning my father asked Danny what he loved most about himself, and Danny said he liked that he was so healthy. My dad told me, "That's sort of how I feel about him, too. A part of me is very clear about the fact that Danny may eventually develop crippling diseases, but I feel like I keep that information in the deep recesses of my consciousness. I'm choosing to focus on the present where Danny is the perfect image of health and vitality. The problem is that because of this, I'm not as careful as I should be. I simply enjoy being with him."

Another Family to Lean On

Danny had a school friend named Zach whose parents, Jack and Robin, took the time to master the details of diabetes. When Danny was at their house, they reminded him to test, supervised his shots, managed his carbohydrates, and made sure the boys stayed active rather than watching television or playing video games. We were incredibly lucky to have such good friends. Robin worked especially hard to educate herself, and this is what she told me about her perspective:

"From my point of view dealing with diabetes is a question of sticking to a schedule and testing a lot. The first time I had Danny, I was apprehensive. Now it's not a big deal. There's medical care nearby, but he's never been sick with me, and we've never needed it. When I have Danny, I test a lot because I don't know the signals that indicate he's high or low. If he's low, I just give him glucose tabs and some carbohydrates. You don't want to overreact and give him too much because then you get a yo-yo effect, and trying to regain control gets impossible. If he's high, though, I'm more concerned. With highs, I go for exercise as well as insulin. Sometimes when they are running around a lot, the concern is getting carbs *into* him."

I asked Robin why she wasn't afraid to be in charge of Danny.

"The thing is, you gave me so much information. I also looked on the Internet and talked to my sister's son who has diabetes. Information alleviates the fear. I can also talk to Danny about what I'm doing. He knows what he needs, and he educates me. At the same time, he's a child and he forgets. When he gets up and comes downstairs in the morning, I don't say, 'Good morning.' I say, 'Have you tested?' and I make sure he does.

"We always do better if he only has a few carbs at night and if I put him to bed at a reasonable number, I know I'm okay. If he's high or low, I get up during the night. I want him to wake up somewhere between eighty and one hundred. If he doesn't, I take it personally.

"Once early on, we were bowling and Danny said, 'I'm feeling low.' I told him to test, and it turned out we hadn't brought his kit. Since we were in the middle of a game, I got him some M&Ms. I could tell he was excited, thinking he was going to eat all of them, but I gave him only five or six because I didn't want him to go too high. Sugar works pretty fast, and I could tell by looking that he was better soon. So we forgot the kit. No one died," she continued. "Jack and I took the kids to my niece's birthday party. The boys had been running around and playing for hours, but when we tested Danny, he was in the high two hundreds. I didn't know about how effective exercise could be at the time, but I had a feeling we should wait instead of going straight for the insulin. We were driving home, and he felt low. When we tested, Danny was seventy-four. It was a good thing I hadn't given him insulin."

"Isn't the food and exercise a lot to deal with?" I asked.

"I see eye-to-eye with your approach to diet. We're a low carb household, too, and this is how we eat anyway. I think it would be much harder for people with junk food in the house. When Danny's coming, I talk to Zach beforehand because I don't want him eating something that Danny can't have. It's not fair. I stock up on a variety of 'nibbles' before Danny comes over, not because of the massive quantities they'll consume, but because I want the boys to have choices. I feel it's better to say, 'Do you want X or Y, rather than eat this…'

"We eat meats and vegetables and cut out pasta. For dinner, we have meatballs and salad or hot dogs and broccoli. The boys eat the same thing. You don't want to create habits now that will make diabetes more difficult as they get older."

She agrees with me about exercise. "It's everything with diabetes. Sometimes I let the boys watch a movie at night, but during the day, they should be active. Exercise is healthy for all children.

"In an emergency, I'd call you because you're very calm. If I couldn't reach you, I'd call your doctor at the numbers you've given me or hit 9-1-1. Actually, I'm not as worried about the risks of diabetes as I am about the way the boys play. They are more likely to crash heads and end up in the ER."

Communicating with Our Doctors

At the end of February, after our second meeting with our new medical team, I wrote our first doctor the following letter:

Dear Dr. C,

I wanted to let you know I am very grateful for the care you've given Danny. Since we last saw you, Danny has had two big changes in insulin needs. During February break, we went to Puerto Rico and Danny went from needing three to five units of insulin per day to needing twelve to fourteen units per day. It was a crazy vacation. Danny's numbers went berserk. We kept adding more and more Humalog and slowly increasing the Lantus to keep up and by the time we left, he was getting shots seven times a day, one at each meal and snack, instead of the usual two or three.

We had one scare when Danny decided to go snorkeling with his dad. It was his first time. He began having trouble with his mask leaking when he and Brian were quite a way offshore. Then Danny reported that he was getting tired and complained that he could barely lift his arms. The two of them decided to head back in. Luckily, Brian is a strong swimmer and hauled Danny in to shore. When my dad and I got to him, he was crying and his head was sagging. When we tested him, his blood sugar level was at sixty-two and after giving him a glucose tab, we had to wait until Danny felt better before we headed back to our place. Danny is a strong swimmer, but they might have been a lot farther out. We all felt shaky because we'd let down our vigilance and the result had been a close call.

When we returned home, Danny went back to acupuncture. He had missed three weeks of treatment, but he immediately went back down to five units of Lantus with one or two extra shots of small amounts of Humalog a day. We breathed a sigh of relief when his blood sugars were in a good range again. Then (I can hardly bear to report this), Danny got the flu and went up to twenty units a day and shots every two hours. A week later, he's better and is now on 6.5 units of Lantus and one or two shots of Humalog in the evening. For the moment, things feel relatively calm. Danny seems healthy and full of energy and the diabetes is again becoming a backdrop rather than center stage news. It has been fourteen months since his diagnosis.

Though we have decided to stay with our new medical team at present, we continue to be very grateful for your care and concern.

Sincerely,

Laura Plunkett

Simplifying Danny's Treatment

Having a child with diabetes doesn't spare you from the other demands of everyday life. I realized one morning that Jessie needed clothes, I had overdue videos to return, our cars needed inspection stickers, and the kids' bike tires were flat. Jessie had an orthodontic appointment, and both kids needed haircuts. There was also food shopping, meal preparation, helping with homework, and shuttling the kids to soccer practice. It was clear to me that I needed to streamline Danny's care if I was going to survive.

In mid-April, fifteen months after diagnosis, Danny's Hemoglobin A1c was 8.3. He was up to eleven units of Lantus in the morning, which gave him a basal dose for twenty-four hours. He was also getting approximately six units of short-acting insulin. Now that he needed insulin at lunch, we sent him to school with five different shots of Humalog in a Tupperware container with the amount labeled on each one and a chart to see which shot he should give himself. It was a lot of work.

I'd seen a pen-like insulin delivery device in a magazine, and I asked our nurse diabetes educator whether this was an option for us. She promptly mailed us a Novopen, which delivers Novolog, an equivalent to Humalog, in incremental units. Now Danny was able to dial up and inject the right amount of insulin without dealing with multiple syringes. Again, we were reminded that if we didn't stay on high alert, our medical team might not take the initiative to tell us about innovations.

Danny was starting to lose weight so we decided to add a few more high-quality carbohydrates to his diet. We encouraged him to eat as much fruit, vegetables, nuts, and whole grains as he wanted and gave him more Novolog at each meal to cover it. I replaced his supplements with a multivitamin with a dark green vegetable base. I found a vitamin for the whole family with many of the recommended ingredients for diabetes control, such as alpha lipoic acid and chromium, and I took Danny off everything else.

In addition, Danny took even more responsibility for his care, testing and giving himself injections during the day while we watched. Brian was doing the middle-of-the-night check, sometimes more than once a night. Although I didn't get out of bed, I woke up, and we figured out what to do together.

At the same time, I was forced to admit that no matter how deeply I cared, I could no longer make the four-hour round trip for acupuncture. I'd initially assumed that Danny's honeymoon would be short-lived but now, in our second year, I found the driving and the toll on our family life too much of a burden. I'd had a problem with my back since I'd ruptured a disc as a teenager and the recent stress had triggered a flare-up which made it extremely uncomfortable to drive. At some point, every caretaker has to respect and accept her limits. At a gut level, I just couldn't make us go anymore.

I was astonished to find that Danny didn't want to stop. He'd grown fond of Bo-In Lee and didn't want to give up our trips. Since I remained convinced that acupuncture kept his body at its highest functioning levels, I assured him I'd find someone just as nice closer to home and that we could continue going out for a meal afterward.

He still didn't want to switch.

I told Danny that I'd heard of an acupuncturist ten minutes from his school. Ra'ufa Clark at Heart of the Rose had been on Dr. Andrew Weil's clinical staff and had taught acupuncture at two respected acupuncture schools. I explained that we could have great adventures near home. I heard myself cajoling, "No traffic. We'll be home before dark," but he just shook his head. In the end, I insisted he had to meet her.

At our first meeting, Ra'ufa was clearly comfortable with children. She had a very gentle style and a less painful technique. She'd done a significant amount of research about juvenile diabetes and explained the Eastern view of Danny's condition that had to do with balancing the functioning of kidneys, lungs, and spleen. Herbs were once again recommended to support these organs.

Though I'd been sure Danny would like her, he complained all the way home. After five or six visits, however, he was laughing and talking with her in a way he never had with the more formal Bo-In Lee. Her treatments didn't affect his body as powerfully as Bo-In Lee's had, perhaps because his diabetes was in a later stage, but ultimately Danny and I were both happier. Ra'ufa became part of our family team and when Danny was sick, I'd spend time on the phone with her, brainstorming ways to make him more comfortable. She always had suggestions for diet or pressure points I should massage.

Unfortunately, Danny started having headaches and stomachaches again. Our family physician did a physical exam and a series of blood tests, ruling out celiac disease, an allergy to gluten. All of them came back normal. I offered to bring Danny back to Bo-In Lee, but it turned out that he'd made the break emotionally and didn't want to return. I didn't argue. Once again, Brian and I had to stand by while Danny was uncomfortable.

Hosting a Juvenile Diabetes Research Foundation Coffee

In June, I hosted my first Juvenile Diabetes Research Foundation coffee. JDRF offers parents the opportunity to meet other parents who are dealing with similar issues. I'd attended several meetings in other towns when Danny was first diagnosed. Now I was eager to meet women in my own community. One Wednesday morning, the four women who came all had girls, now teenagers, who had been diagnosed with diabetes as toddlers or young children.

Although they'd been dealing with diabetes far longer than I had, the best part of the meeting was how much we all had in common. I described Danny's wide fluctuations in blood sugar levels, and they all nodded knowingly. I described our difficulties traveling and all of them acknowledged having trouble taking trips also. I talked about being anxious all the time and discovered two of them were on anti-anxiety medication. As they spoke, I realized we all got up in the middle of the night to test our kids and had too many doctors' appointments. We all felt that no one understood what we were going though and agreed that although the passage of time made it easier, it never got easy. We would all do anything for our children.

I often scolded myself for worrying too much, but I discovered that these lovely, high-functioning, intelligent women worried as much, if not more, than I did. In some cases, families had given up traveling, and the mothers still went along on every one of their children's field trips. Later I was able to call Brian at work and reassure him that our family was mirrored by every one of these families, no matter how long they'd been coping.

I was struck by the way these women had managed to find support and a degree of freedom. Many families who had met each other at JDRF functions or diabetes camp weekends had teamed up. They watched each other's children and turned to one another in hard times. Their children slept over at each other's houses, secure in the presence of a knowledgeable adult.

I knew that worrying about the future was a waste of time, but I also learned that three of the four children were already suffering from complications caused by their diabetes. I didn't want to know the grim details, but one had a circulatory problem and two had problems with kidney functioning.

I didn't tell Brian that.

Coping with the Croup

The night before his last day of third grade, Danny came into our room at one in the morning, holding his throat and whispering that he couldn't breathe. We'd checked him an hour earlier and his blood sugar level had been in the 300s, so now we suspected croup and put him into the steam of our shower. Both our kids had been through bouts of croup as toddlers, but this seemed far more severe. I reached our primary care physician at home and when Dr. Horowitz said it might be asthma, which is reaching epidemic proportions in our area, I felt a wave of nausea at the thought of Danny having yet another disease. I had to sit on the edge of the bed and breathe deeply in order to fight off a feeling of panic.

Dr. Horowitz suggested taking Danny to the emergency room. I looked at Brian holding Danny in the shower and realized that I'd had so little sleep during the week that I was weak with fatigue. Brian and I had fallen into a pattern of staying up late so that we could have time together, but after getting up for

Danny during the night, we both still woke up at six. I felt as if I might faint. I splashed my face with water and got dressed, but I couldn't find any hidden resources. I was nauseous and dizzy, and my son couldn't breathe. I pictured getting to the hospital and not being able to function. I'd never had that fear about myself before.

I volunteered to stay home with Jessie, not wanting to admit that I was at the end of my strength. In those few moments of negotiation, Danny's breathing got even worse. Now we felt we needed an adult with Brian in the car in case Danny stopped breathing completely *and* someone home with Jessie. We woke my dad out of a sound sleep, and he was at our door in five minutes. He and Brian took Danny to the hospital while I called the ER to warn them that they were coming.

I dialed the emergency room our doctor recommended and leaned my head against the wall while the nurse on duty told me that all the examining rooms were full, but they'd try to "fit him in." I told her Danny had diabetes and she said, "Yeahhh?" with an attitude. Her unspoken "So what?" alarmed me. I felt uneasy about sending Danny there, especially after our previous experience.

On impulse, I called a children's hospital closer to our house. The nurse who answered said there were only two patients currently waiting. She would immediately inform the doctor of Danny's diabetes and have a respirator waiting for him. We began the registration process over the phone. I gave the nurse the information she needed and then redirected Brian over his cell phone.

After I hung up, I staggered upstairs. How could I have let myself get so overtired that I could barely move? What kind of mother didn't go to the hospital with her son? Yet, I was too bone tired even for self-reproach. Despite my fear about Danny's condition, after I checked on Jessie, I slept.

As it turned out, I wasn't needed. Danny was on a respirator seven minutes after he left the house. Fortunately, his x-ray revealed croup rather than asthma. The ER doctor got in contact with our new endocrinology team in order to check the impact of a steroid called Decadron, which makes children insulin resistant for five days. They decided Danny desperately needed this medication and started him on it immediately. He and Brian were home by four o'clock and back to sleep soon afterwards.

In the morning, Danny felt remarkably well though his blood sugar was over 300. He cheerily announced that he could still go to the party on his last day of school, but the doctor had warned us that, with his blood sugars bound to run high, he needed to be tested every two hours. If he developed ketones, he'd have to go back to the hospital. When I told him we didn't dare let him go, he cried. His birthday ruined and now this. At that moment, I felt as if my heart was breaking.

Nonetheless, I was relieved to have him home. For the next five days, we tested Danny every two hours around the clock and gave him additional insulin as needed. Danny was often in the 300s and 400s. On the second day, he went from sixteen units a day to forty units! It was scary and exhausting, and the stress from trying to avoid another hospitalization was ridiculous. We were guessing how much insulin to give him, and, truthfully, even his doctors didn't have a clue what would work in this situation. If a child tests over 240, he's not supposed to exercise, but exercise is one of the best ways to fight insulin resistance. I tried to get Danny to play games with me, but his high numbers left him feeling so tired that he just lay on the couch.

It was a long, sad, first week of summer.

Eventually, however, the Decadron wore off, and Danny's numbers stabilized. Soon he was up and running through the neighborhood, playing basketball, and riding his bike. Breathing a sigh of relief, we realized, to our surprise, that no matter how hard and scary sick days were, the rest of the time we'd begun to think of Danny as well.

CHAPTER 7

▼

The Second Sixth
Months

Danny's Two Weeks at Farm Camp

Danny left for Hawthorne Valley Farm Camp at the end of June. I'd spoken with Gisela, the camp nurse, several times over the winter. She was nervous, but excited to learn how to care for him. She agreed that it was extremely important for Danny to be able to go to a regular camp instead of feeling limited by his disease. I knew I was taking a calculated risk, but I felt confident. Gisela was an experienced nurse. Danny was already very independent and trustworthy. I saw the glint in Danny's eye. He didn't want to go to diabetes camp. He wanted to live on a farm. Any worry on our part would be worth it.

I spent the better part of two weeks ordering supplies, making lists, preparing emergency protocols, assembling informational packets for the staff, adjusting our daily log to his camp schedule, teaching Danny to be as self-sufficient as he'd need to be, and warding off the advice of people who were afraid we'd live to regret this. Dr. J helped us change Danny's insulin doses to match his anticipated increase in activity level. She told us how to raise his bedtime numbers so that the staff wouldn't need to test him at night.

Then Brian and I drove Danny to New York.

After camp orientation, Brian went home with the parents of one of Danny's camp friends while I stayed at a nearby bed and breakfast until Gisela felt confident. During the first two days, I met with her four times and spoke with different staff members on several occasions. Gisela and I agreed that when I went home, we'd speak on the phone at seven thirty each morning and eight thirty each night to decide on insulin doses.

By the time I left, Danny was all set. Gisela told me he took his shots right in his seat in the dining hall. When the kids wanted to know, "What is that? Does it hurt?" he'd say, "It's a shot. It doesn't really hurt that much after you get used to it." She said the kids were curious and friendly. I drove home feeling optimistic.

When I got home, I felt both free and pressured. How could I fit everything I wanted to do into two precious weeks? How could I have time alone with Brian and Jessie and still see all the friends I'd neglected? Should I tackle all my unfinished tasks or indulge myself? Ultimately I did a little of everything. Brian went to jujitsu while Jessie and I went to the movies and to a late night women's soccer game. I went into Danny's room with trash bags and really cleaned it up. We ate whenever we were hungry instead of according to Danny's strict schedule, though we didn't change our diet much. Brian and I went camping in Vermont one weekend while Jessie stayed with my sister.

Still, even with Danny three and one-half hours away, I was acutely aware of being "on call." Gisela called at seven thirty every morning so I couldn't sleep late. She called me between eight thirty and nine at night so I had to be available every evening. If issues came up, we also conferred during the day. Often she'd apologize, "Oh, it wasn't a good day," meaning that Danny's blood sugars had fluctuated wildly. I had to reassure her that it was the same at home and that no matter how hard she tried, this disease was just not predictable.

By the end of the second week, I yearned to stop being the one in charge. I made plans to eat out with my friend Amanda. As a pediatric nurse, Amanda understood our situation. She had been a very good friend, calling to check on us and cooking us meals. I was looking forward to time alone with her. I asked Brian to take Gisela's call. Before I left, I reminded him to stay where he could hear the phone.

At a quarter of nine, my cell phone rang at the restaurant table. It was Gisela, flustered because she'd been calling our house for fifteen minutes and no one had picked up. I stepped outside to spare Amanda the details and spent the next ten minutes choosing how much insulin Danny should have before bed. I rejoined Amanda with a smile, but I felt defeated.

When I got home, Brian and Jessie were stretched out on the couch, happily watching a video. When Brian looked up, I could see him suddenly remembering that he'd been commissioned to talk to Gisela. Then he noticed the flashing light on the answering machine and started to panic. He hadn't heard the phone ring.

"I never talked to the nurse," he said. I told him I'd spoken to her from the restaurant. He looked bewildered. "Why did you take your cell phone to the restaurant?" I just looked at him until we both acknowledged in silence that one moment's lapse in attention could cost us everything.

Jessie enjoyed being an only child for two weeks. We talked about every subject under the sun, and I could tell she loved our relaxed time together. Yet, she wrote Danny every single day, sometimes more than once, and several times, she biked into town to find special cards to send him. When my mother asked if she was looking forward to Danny's homecoming, she said she wasn't.

"It's really hard when he's here," she explained. "Things feel different."

"But," my mother reported, "she was talking about his diabetes, not him."

We drove to New York to bring Danny home on Saturday and met with Gisela before we saw him. She described Danny as one of the most energetic children at the camp and said he had no trouble making friends or fitting in. In fact, when Danny gave himself shots, she described how the kids often gathered around and asked him questions. Although Danny was the camp's first child with diabetes, she said she'd gladly have him again next year.

Brian said, "It must have been exhausting taking care of him," and although she'd eaten all her meals at his table and checked his blood sugars five to six times a day, she reassured us, "This has been a great learning experience for me. I want to make this camp the kind of place kids with special needs can come." We were blessed to have found her.

When we finally located Danny, he was covered in mosquito bites and smelled like a cow barn. Nevertheless, he was very happy. All the way home in the car, he told us about his adventures, including sleeping outdoors without a tent, hiking up a mountain, riding horses without a saddle, swimming in a lake, and mucking out the cow barn. He never mentioned his diabetes, Gisela, or the food.

Reflexology

While Danny was away, I met a woman at a party who practiced foot reflexology, which is a form of acupressure. Rather than use needles on the meridians of the body as they do in acupuncture, Ann Wettlaufer massaged points on people's feet and thereby affected their health and well-being. She overheard me discussing Danny with a friend and before I left that night, said that she felt drawn to work with him. She offered to reduce her fee significantly for three sessions to see if she could make a difference in his insulin needs.

I followed up our conversation by calling several friends who knew Ann. Each one raved about her ability as a healer and thought I should take her up on her offer. Danny was still troubled by stomachaches and headaches, and I was looking for help with those symptoms. I scheduled his first appointment for the beginning of July.

Now Danny was protesting. He was on summer time and determined to stay that way until I explained that he could read *Harry Potter* through his "foot massages." Then he decided we should go *now*. Ann had a diagram on the wall of her office and showed him his pancreas and digestive tract with the corresponding points on his feet. She explained to him that, like acupuncture, her work was designed to stimulate certain organs in his body. He seemed intrigued and asked a couple of questions. Then he removed his shoes and socks, lay down on the table, and disappeared into his book.

After the first session, Danny began having a series of lows and rapidly required less insulin. Two days after the third session, he had gone from twenty-four units in twenty-four hours to twelve units in the same time period. Danny also stopped complaining about aches and pains.

It seemed incredibly far-fetched that foot reflexology could affect Danny in this way, but it was noninvasive, Danny liked it, and it was helping. Not only was he feeling better, but also I felt more lighthearted. The fact that Danny and I were actually doing something besides simply increasing his insulin filled me with a sense of purpose, which I seemed to need. For me, resignation was far more demoralizing than going to appointments. Ann agreed she'd see Danny again in the fall. His improvement lasted through most of August.

We got the results of Danny's eighteen-month Hemoglobin A1c test that reflected his blood sugar control in April, May, and June. It was 8.1. Our nurse diabetes educator attributed the rise to the Decadron Danny had taken for croup. She wrote that we should just keep doing what we were doing. All I can say about our response is that we resolved to try harder.

Talking about Death with Danny

"Mom, what happens if I get so low that I faint?" Danny asked. We were in the car, on the way to a doctor's appointment.

"Then I either squirt some frosting into your mouth or I give you a shot of glucagon, your blood sugar goes up and you wake up," I replied.

"Well, what happens if you're not there?"

"Someone will call 9-1-1, and the EMTs will take care of you."

"What if I'm all alone and no one's there?"

"You'll stay in a coma until someone finds you and calls 9-1-1."

"What if no one finds me?"

"Then you would die, Danny."

"Oh, bummer!"

One Week at Family Diabetes Camp

In mid-July, our family headed north to Sebago Lake in Maine where Camp Sunshine serves the families of children who have life-threatening illnesses, from cancer to lupus to diabetes. Each disease gets a separate week all to itself. The camp's philosophy is that the families of sick children need support and rest, and to fill that need, the camp offers counseling and parent groups as well as camp activities and time for relaxation. Families are selected by lottery and all expenses are paid by donors who give fifteen hundred dollars to sponsor each family. Along with the forty families who are chosen, seventy volunteers give up a week of their summer to insure a carefree and nurturing experience.

Brian and I finally had the energy to reach out to other families, and we were interested in seeing how other families were coping. All of us were excited to have this opportunity.

As I began to pack, it occurred to me that I should check the camp's menu to see what foods I should bring. The head cook read me a typical day's menu. For breakfast, they served Cocoa Puffs, Fruit Loops, and Danish pastry along with plain yogurt and fresh fruit. Lunches and dinners offered similar high carbohydrate, high-sugar temptations. Brian and I tried to prepare the kids for what to expect, but after hearing about the food, Danny decided he didn't want to go. Then he changed his mind.

"At first I didn't want to go to Camp Sunshine because my mother found out there was junk food there, like pizza and cookies and all that kind of stuff, and it's not good for me," he told my mother. "But now I do because the whole family's going to eat whatever I eat and we're just going to eat what we can. We're going to bring food with us so, if I'm hungry, I can go back to the room for more."

We arrived on Sunday afternoon. We were met in the parking lot by at least ten smiling, yellow-shirted volunteers, who gathered around our van. They brought our bags up to our second-floor apartment overlooking a volleyball court. Each family had its own suite with a bedroom, a full bath, a kitchen with refrigerator and microwave, and a living room with a futon couch and a bunk bed. The camp boasted a miniature golf course, tetherball, a soccer field, a climbing wall, shuffleboard, a computer room, and a lakefront area with paddle boats, kayaks, and canoes. There was an arts and crafts center, a game room, and an indoor pool, all state-of-the-art and brand new.

As we met other families that night, we were thrilled. We couldn't believe how lucky we were to have been given this opportunity.

From that first evening, both kids were scheduled for a succession of activities. They were both in the nine-to-twelve age group with great counselors. Danny's caretaker was a nursing student named Mike, who had only four children in his care. Mike was in charge of all Danny's diabetes needs at camp when we weren't with him; Brian and I could fully relax during the day. There were nursing supervisors as well as an endocrinologist in residence that week.

Brian and I had a very busy schedule. Mornings, we had optional group counseling with all the other parents. Afternoons, the adults took part in cooperative games, archery, swimming, and other activities. Evenings, there was a talent show, a masquerade ball, and a karaoke night for families.

The social worker who led our counseling group had been doing this work for over twenty years. She facilitated about forty-five of us and made it look easy. Everyone warmed to her immediately. Her first question was, "How many of you are sleeping through the night?" When we all burst into laughter, she pointed out that everyone in the room already had something in common.

For the first time Brian and I caught an intimate look at how other couples were coping with the demands of this illness. When the social worker asked how many of us felt anger, depression, guilt, or anxiety, every hand went up. We listened to people reveal a huge range of experiences. The husbands of several women had walked out of their marriages soon after their child's diagnosis and never looked back. Some of the parents had not gotten a babysitter since their children's illness, including one couple who hadn't had a night out in nine years.

Some couples seemed to work well together, but in a large percentage of the families, diabetes had driven people apart, especially in circumstances where the burden of care giving fell primarily upon the mother. Some fathers regretted that long hours at work kept them from being an integral part of family life; other fathers admitted that their own denial had distanced them from what was happening at home. Many parents continued to feel very angry that this had happened to their family and struggled to contain it.

A majority felt that no one understood what they were going through, including their extended families. We heard anecdotes of grandparents who refused to learn about the disease or decided to continue to spend time only with the healthy child. In many cases, when children with diabetes visited or stayed with relatives, including ex-husbands, they were overindulged and their diabetes regimen thrown out the window.

I was especially interested when someone started talking about how family and friends would ask, "Why are you so uptight?" or "Why are you so stressed out about this?" as if after some period of time, parents should loosen up and go with the flow. No one had said those things to me, but I often said them to myself. Clearly, it was time to give that up.

When the counselor asked, "How many of you moms feel you always have to be the bad guy?" Brian was surprised I didn't raise my hand. He told me later that he thought I often had that role, but I pointed out that even though I was usually the one who laid down the law, he supported me. Suddenly it was clear that what I minded most wasn't being the bad guy, but always feeling in charge, and though I knew it couldn't be helped, I still resented it. Sitting around after lunch, sharing our reactions, Brian and I realized again how much we missed having uninterrupted time to talk.

The pharmaceutical sales representatives who set up tables in the hallway were very helpful. Our family learned about the latest technology, including the pump. Danny got a private demonstration, and he was enthusiastic until he saw how the plastic catheter was inserted under the skin. At that point, Danny vehemently said that he didn't want anything attached to his body, no matter how convenient it might be.

We also attended a lecture given by the visiting endocrinologist. After he gave us an update on the latest research, a woman raised her hand and said that she'd heard that children who fall into comas from extremely low blood sugars don't die. Was that true? The endocrinologist said that in many cases the child's pancreas releases glucagon and the child revives on his own. I hadn't known that. In the dining hall, I explained that to Danny.

His response? "Cool! Let's get lunch."

Our only problem at camp came at mealtimes. The food was served cafeteria style, and Danny had to walk past all of it on the way to a table. This meant that at every meal he was tempted by items that Brian and I considered to be of no nutritional value. Of course, Danny absolutely couldn't pass up the slices of pizza, the macaroni and cheese, the chicken nuggets, or the brownies when almost every child in the line had a tray full of them. We let him choose one or two of those foods along with vegetables and salad.

His total carbohydrates per meal went from forty to sixty to eighty, and before our eyes, we saw the effects of sugar and white flour and fried food. For the first time, one unit of Novolog only covered ten grams of carbohydrate whereas at home, one unit usually handled twenty to thirty grams. We pointed this out to Mike, Danny's nurse, who said, "How come they didn't teach me that in school?"

One night there was a camp-out in tents around a fire. The counselors served S'mores as the bedtime snack, which consist of two graham crackers filled with a marshmallow and a chocolate bar. The kids stayed up until midnight and were up again at five in the morning. I warned Mike that Danny's numbers would be high, since lack of sleep always drove his numbers up. Midmorning, Mike came running over to me with the news that Danny was 399.

I asked, "Didn't I call it?"

"Not only did you call it," he said, "but all the kids are running just as high and all the nurses are noticing the change."

On Thursday in group counseling, Brian and I brought up the fact that Danny was now on twice his usual amount of insulin. Many parents were seeing the same thing, but not one person in the room seemed to agree with us that complex carbohydrates, whole grains, fruits, and vegetables were an important part of the diet. Several parents cautioned us that restricting a child's diet, or keeping him from eating "typical" foods, would lead to eating disorders. Another said that it was important "to let kids be kids." When my husband wondered aloud why people thought an emphasis on healthy food would create more problems than eating junk food, the nutritionist ended the discussion by saying that the most important thing is to avoid creating serious eating issues by letting kids eat what they want.

She repeated the mantra: "A carb is a carb."

For the first time that week, Brian and I walked away from a meeting feeling isolated and alone. I felt like the odd one out, so shaky that I thought about going home. To my surprise, two women immediately came up to us to say that they fed their children diets similar to Danny's, but that they hadn't dared to say it openly. What a relief! Our families became allies, especially at mealtimes.

Despite the food issues, we loved the camp. Danny was the happiest of us all. He loved hanging out with kids like him, he loved the constant activity, he loved Mike and all his counselors, and he loved that he was eating food he never got at home. Jessie made friends with a girl with diabetes and wanted to come back next year when she would be eligible for the teen group. Camp Sunshine was a very positive experience, and we agreed we'd be lucky if we were chosen again.

"Camp Sunshine was a totally normal camp," Jessie told my mother, "except that there were nurses around and my parents. We were very lucky because other people volunteered to pay for us. Just because you have diabetes, you aren't any different from anyone else so the kids with diabetes did everything with the regular kids. I made friends with a girl my age who wore a pump. I'd never seen one before. She didn't wear her pump into the lake because if it fell off, she might lose it. The only bad thing was the food was very unhealthy."

Sometime after our visit, the camp began to evaluate the fat, sugar, and grain content of their food program. They planted a large garden and increased the availability of fruits, vegetables, and whole grains as they moved toward a healthier meal plan. We were excited to hear the news.

The Diabetes Diet War

In July of 2003, after we returned from Camp Sunshine, I came across an article by Dara Mayers in a magazine called *Health & Medicine*.

"The nutrition advice given to most diabetics might be killing them," she begins, criticizing the *Diabetes Food and Nutrition Bible*, published by the American Diabetes Association. "Grains, beans, and starchy vegetables form the foundation of the Diabetes Food Pyramid. The message is to eat more of these foods than from any of the other food groups." This message is strongly supported by many doctors and nutritionists and promoted to seventeen million Americans with diabetes.

I'd had no idea that a high-carbohydrate diet was the subject of heated debate in the diabetes community. Mayers quotes Scott King, editor-in-chief of *Diabetes Interview* magazine as saying, "It is the most controversial aspect of diabetes treatment today." She also quotes Lois Jovanovic, chief scientific officer of the Sansum Medical Research Institute in Santa Barbara, California, who goes so far as to call this conventional nutritional advice "malpractice."

Historically, Mayers says, the pyramid was created to combat the cardiovascular problems that often plague people with diabetes. As cholesterol and fat were linked to heart disease, experts recommended a low-fat diet and increased the amount of carbohydrates included in the diet to fill the void. In 1994, Nathaniel Clark, national vice president for clinical affairs at the ADA, proclaimed that people with diabetes could eat anything, including sugar itself. "There is no longer a diabetic diet. People with diabetes eat the exact same foods as anyone else," Mayers quotes him as saying. "We do not believe there is any harm in eating carbohydrates."

The ADA claims that, "a diet that is very low in carbohydrates is significantly higher in protein and in fat, and there are specific risks to people with diabetes from high-protein diets in regard to kidney disease and from high-fat diets in regard to cardiovascular disease." Places like the Joslin Diabetes Center in Boston continue to recommend that 45 to 60 percent of calories eaten by people with diabetes come from carbohydrates. The ADA Web site and all of its literature continue to encourage people with diabetes to make starches "the centerpiece of the meal."

Mayers counters this view with the opinions of Dr. Richard Bernstein, whose book, *Dr. Bernstein's Diabetes Solution,* had so impressed me, and Lois Jovanovic, who strongly disagree. They consider diabetes to be a disease of "carbohydrate intolerance." Mayers' article gave several case studies in which low-carb diets not only stabilized blood sugar levels in people with diabetes, but also reduced the patient's cholesterol profile, a finding supported by studies of dieters following the Atkins low-carb regimen. Frank Hu, an associate professor of nutrition and epidemiology at the Harvard School of Public Health, also believes that lower-carb diets can be beneficial to some people with diabetes, but only if carbohydrates are replaced with "healthy fats," such as the mono- and polyunsaturated fats found in olive oil, nuts, and avocados.

Mayers is hopeful that this new data will have an impact. She quotes ADA board member Barbara Kahn, a physician and diabetes expert at Harvard Medical School, as saying that, "the ADA is responsive to new scientific data and is likely to incorporate this information into new dietary guidelines with a lower proportion of carbohydrates."

Yes!!!!!

Feelings of Mastery, Finally

By August, I was feeling stronger and healthier though it's hard to quantify something as elusive as a feeling of well-being. Our lives were running so much more smoothly that I became aware that my anxiety level didn't always fit what was happening. I'd be feeling fine, but if the slightest problem arose—a low or very high blood sugar, an injury, or even too much happening at once—my adrenaline would kick in. I'd get a feeling of dread and feel shaky and scared. Even when I slept, I was on constant alert.

Ra'ufa Clark, Danny's acupuncturist, suggested that my biggest priority should be sleep. Brian and I had been waking up, sometimes as many as three times a night. She pointed out that interrupted sleep might be contributing to my nervous tension and anxiety so on our vacation, Brian let me sleep from midnight to nine in the morning. He got up at night without waking me and gave Danny his morning insulin at seven o'clock. Then he'd come back to bed and doze while the kids read books and played in the living room. Because Brian's energy level was much higher than mine was, he could maintain this pace indefinitely. I'd tried to keep up with him without realizing the toll it was taking.

By the end of our time away, I was a lot less anxious and a lot more cheerful. I found myself laughing at things that would have bothered me at home. Everyone noticed that Mommy was feeling better, especially me.

When we returned home, we were busy again, but I still felt looser and more relaxed than at any time since Danny's diagnosis. I noticed I'd stopped thinking of myself as a person with a sick child. Everyone has problems, and Danny's diabetes was becoming just one of the problems our family faced.

Jessie had taken a babysitting and first aid course and began sitting for other families as well as for Danny. Brian and I were delighted. Now, when we returned, after leaving Danny with Jessie for short periods of time, it was nice to hear both kids protesting that we should've stayed away longer. More and more we trusted Jessie's judgment and her competence in an emergency.

When I asked her about babysitting, she was nonchalant. "He tests his own blood and gives himself shots. If I put him to bed, I stay up. I'm not nervous that something might happen, like him falling into a coma."

She looked thoughtful. "It would be kind of exciting, actually. First, I'd make sure he wasn't just sleeping. If I couldn't wake him up, I'd call the hospital and if they said to, I'd give him a shot from the emergency glucagon kit. I'd call you from the ambulance on your cell phone. I'd take care of him first because it's more important that I make sure he's safe than that you know what's happening. It's kind of impossible that would happen though, unless he was asleep, because he's good now at catching himself when he's low."

It was true. Danny was reporting his lows now and noticing how he felt, but I was aware that Jessie was the one that caught the symptoms we missed. I told her so.

"I know that when he's low he gets grumpy, he cries, or he seems tired and I'm almost one hundred percent right," she said. "When he acts up, he's usually low. When he's low, he cries when just a little thing is wrong. He thinks it's never going to turn out right, like, he might be hungry and think we're not going to give him enough food, though we always do. If I don't know he's low, it makes me angry that he's such a wimp. Sometimes it seems like he doesn't trust us. Then when he takes a glucose tab, he is back to himself again."

As our school schedule kicked in, I offered Danny the choice of Bo-In Lee or Ra'ufa for acupuncture, or Ann for reflexology, knowing that with those choices he couldn't go wrong. Danny chose to alternate. He wanted to continue seeing Ra'ufa because our visits included dinner and a trip to the toy store. He liked seeing Ann because he could read, and he liked being free by four thirty in the afternoon when he could still play outside. His decision was fine with me. His reasons were based on an eight-year-old perspective, but I wanted him to feel like he had some freedom in his choice of treatments.

In September, Ann asked to see Danny three days in a row. She hadn't seen him since July, and she wanted to get him "balanced" before she started seeing him twice a month. Danny did homework and read Archie comic books during his sessions. Ann gave him coloring book handouts of his digestive system, his endocrine system, and his foot reflexes, and he read them all with interest.

Danny had been starting the day with fourteen units of Lantus, adding about four units of Novolog at each meal and sometimes during the night. At this level of insulin, the honeymoon appeared over. However, after the first of Ann's treatments, Danny started into what Brian and I called "freefall." Danny quickly went down to ten units of Lantus to start the day, with only one or two units of Novolog at meals. A week after his third session, we noticed that his insulin needs were rising again, but not nearly as fast and as far as they had fallen.

In some cases, it was clear to us which factors determined Danny's blood sugar levels and insulin needs. Carbohydrates, and to a lesser degree, protein raised his sugars. Prolonged exercise dropped them. Exercise with adrenaline, like an intense soccer game, briefly raised them. Lack of sleep brought them up, and a burst of insulin from his pancreas brought them down. Growth spurts, fevers, and stress raised them for long periods of time.

Now another pattern seemed to be emerging. Bo-In Lee had spoken of "organ balance," a body's way of functioning at an optimum level. Initially, we'd seen his attempt to introduce balance set off Danny's honeymoon. Later he'd realigned this balance after each illness. Now Ann had twice created a situation where Danny's numbers dropped after, in her words, she "restructured the flow of his energy and stimulated his organ functioning." No one in conventional medicine had ever mentioned this was possible, but we could see the benefits right before our eyes.

Personally, I was glad to have both Ra'ufa and Ann involved in Danny's care. It can feel very lonely, even with a supportive husband, to carry so much responsibility. Having other women listen to my concerns and work with me in caring for Danny gave me a feeling of direction. Instead of standing alone, I felt like I had companions on the path I was traveling. I knew I could call on either woman at any time, and I felt safer knowing that if something went wrong, they'd be there for us.

Brian turned forty-one in mid-September, and as we entered our favorite breakfast spot to celebrate with friends and family, I noticed how smooth our routine had become. In order to get the children to school on time, we'd had to leave our house by quarter of seven. Our morning routine, a shot of Lantus, a blood glucose test, Chinese herbs, and a multivitamin along with the usual lunch and backpack preparation, went smoothly. Entering a restaurant was no longer anxiety-producing. I knew the amount of carbohydrates Danny would probably order, the right amount of short-acting Novolog to give, and that there would be sugarless maple syrup on the table. When Danny ordered pancakes, Brian and I met eyes and said "three units" at the same moment. That was the only discussion necessary.

Amazing! And it only took us twenty months.

Our Second Halloween

Halloween felt different to all of us this time. I was surprised when a neighbor approached me two weeks before the holiday to tell me she already had Danny's Halloween gift. She asked what costume he'd be wearing so that she could identify him. A second neighbor told me Jessie had reminded her to get something without sugar for Danny and she asked if I would give her some suggestions.

Two days before Halloween, I went to the drugstore and bought silly string, a skull, a glow stick, a slinky, and other small items. On Halloween Day, when I made rounds of the neighborhood with my basket of "treats," I discovered that at least half of the people I approached had already gotten Danny something special. The others were happy to take something to give him. Several women asked me about Danny's health, and it felt good to be able to say that although it was still a full-time job, we were settling into it.

Last October I felt raw, worried, and vulnerable as I went door-to-door. I struggled with how to answer questions without crying. I felt awkward, as if I were doing something weird. This year, I was more comfortable and my neighborhood no longer felt like a place where my son didn't fit in.

At our neighborhood bonfire Halloween night, Danny ate two no-carbohydrate chocolate bars which I'd given him and two regular candy bars, then spent the rest of the night showing his friends all the cool "treats" he'd gotten. With some additional insulin, his blood sugar stayed under control. That night I overheard Danny telling a friend Halloween was his favorite holiday.

Brian had told the kids that he'd buy their candy at ten cents apiece. Laughing, he had encouraged them to go trick-or-treating with king-sized pillowcases. When both kids returned with huge sacks full of candy, Brian lived to regret his offer.

We had a happy Halloween, but for the next two days, Danny's blood sugars ran in the 300s no matter what we did. We couldn't figure out what was happening. I was walking by Danny's room when I heard Jessie asking Danny, "What do you have in your hand? I won't tell Mom."

"Well, you better tell both of us, Danny," I said, walking in. Danny looked sheepish. We cracked up laughing. "Let's not drag this out," I suggested as Jessie and I lay on his bed, waiting for him to open his fist. When he did, there was a partially melted Reese's Cup puddled in his palm.

I asked if he'd been eating his Halloween candy and he replied, "Just a few." That's when I noticed the candy-filled pillowcase beside his bookcase. Brian and I had gone out Saturday night and forgotten to confiscate Danny's loot.

I told Danny two things that occurred to me immediately. First, I reminded him that his blood sugars told his father and me how much insulin to give him, and that if we didn't know that he'd eaten candy, we couldn't properly adjust the dose. I explained that if we raised his dose because his blood sugar was high and he didn't eat another candy bar, he could have a serious low.

"This family's a team," I said, "and we have to know what you're eating in order to keep you safe. There really isn't any room for sneaking food, Danny. It's too dangerous." Then I told him that everyone cheats on his or her goals for themselves, and that his father and I knew there'd be times when he felt he simply had to eat something sweet. "Those are the times you have to trust us enough to come and tell us so we can figure out the right insulin dose. You can eat that piece of candy in your hand," I added, giving him a hug, "and then we'll add insulin."

To my surprise, Danny came downstairs a minute later, dumped the candy in the trash, and washed his sticky hand.

"You can have one that isn't melted," I said.

"I don't need a piece of candy right now," he replied, and went outside to play.

The Be-A-Great-Athlete Approach

In October, we received the results of Danny's twenty-one-month Hemoglobin A1c blood test, reflecting his blood sugar control for July, August, and September. Despite our best efforts, the number was 7.8. I called my aunt Barbara, a primary care physician, and asked for her opinion. She said that if it were her child, she wouldn't rest until she got the number under seven. She considered 7.8 too high and suggested we try a new insulin regimen or a new doctor.

Several days later, I found myself at my friend Christine's house, bemoaning the fact that no matter how carefully we monitored Danny's food and calculated his doses, we still couldn't seem to control the outcome. Danny's blood sugars had been very inconsistent at night, and I was tired of dealing with it. I was sharing my discouragement with Christine when, with a light in her eyes, she said, "Let's make a plan." Caught up in her enthusiasm, by the end of the next hour I had a page of ideas to bring home to my family. I did research on the Internet and called a family meeting. I'd decided to start appealing to Danny as an athlete and soccer player.

I had my presentation all planned.

"You had a great soccer season, Danny," I began. "You've been chosen for the top team in the spring. I know you're excited that Dad's going to be your coach again. At the same time, it's dangerous for you to keep playing with numbers that are too low or too high. We need to keep you even when you play. Dad and I are considering letting both you and Jessie go to sports camp for two weeks this summer, but if you're going to keep your body in top form, we have to make some changes in how you handle your diabetes."

Danny was listening intently.

"I've been researching how athletes with diabetes in the NFL, NHL, and NBA manage their health." At this point, I pulled out a sheaf of color printouts with the biographies of a number of well-known professional athletes and spread them on the table. Danny was amazed to see that so many of them had diabetes. Then, I stretched the truth.

"This is what these players do to keep in top shape," I explained, though their diabetes regimens weren't included in their biographies. "First, you have to learn to estimate your blood sugars. From now on, Dad and I are going to ask you to guess what your blood sugar is before each test," I said. "Even if at first you're not good at it, we think you can get a better sense of whether you're in the high or low range by listening to your body." I'd come up with this idea after finding out that dogs can be trained to sense high and low blood sugars in their owners. If a dog could sense blood sugars in a person, why couldn't a person learn to do it for himself?

I went on, "Two, you have to exercise every day."

I said this because Danny didn't want to play any winter sports, saying he wanted time to be home and hang out with his friends. "If you're going to have level blood sugars, we need to pick some activity for you to do every day without an argument." He and Jessie immediately began generating ideas, including buying a treadmill and a cross-trainer. Their solutions were too expensive, but both of them seemed excited about the plan.

"Three." I continued, "You have to get a solid night's sleep." Of course, Brian and I were hoping we'd get one too.

"The goal is to have good blood sugars while you sleep so your body can rest and regenerate," I explained. "We want to see whether your nighttime blood sugars become more stable if you cut out all carbohydrates at dinner and bedtime snack." I saw alarm on Danny's face. "Don't worry. You'll still have carbs at breakfast, lunch, and three snacks. And Dad and I will eat the same food you do for dinner."

I assumed this would elicit a huge protest, but Danny replied, "OK, I'll go as low-carb as I can." His only request was that he could still have ketchup and salad dressing. To my surprise, Jessie said she'd do it too. Everyone agreed we might as well start right away. I ended our meeting, feeling hopeful again. As with any chronic disease, you have to keep generating renewed enthusiasm or you settle into ruts without noticing how lax you've become. Now at least we had a plan and no one was complaining.

By the beginning of December, we'd put some of my "athlete" ideas into practice at home. Danny was estimating his blood sugars regularly and tended to be within thirty points most of the time. He was more accurate with lows than highs, and he had trouble sensing the difference between 150 and 300, but he was focusing more on how his body felt. Exercise was still a bit haphazard, but he and I created a routine of sit-ups, push-ups, and aerobics that lasted about ten minutes, and sometimes Jessie, Danny, and I did it together several times in a row.

The best part was that Danny was having significantly lower numbers at dinner and bedtime. He was averaging only twenty carbohydrates after four o'clock, eating mostly meat with ketchup or sauce, vegetables, salad, and cheese for dinner. We had loosened our no-artificial-sweetener policy and gave him sugar-free Jell-O at bedtime, which he loved.

The results were stunning. Not only were his numbers better at night, but his body seemed to be handling carbohydrates more efficiently during the day. **His two-week blood sugar average dropped from 180 to 140, and as it happened, three months later his Hemoglobin A1c reading went from 7.8 to 6.8.** This new plan required more forethought and creative cooking, with some of our favorite meals being sorely missed, but it felt worth it. As we adjusted to those lower numbers, Brian and I continued to test him after midnight, but we were hopeful that soon we'd feel confident enough to sleep through the night.

Losing Faith in Our Second Medical Team

Two weeks after the beginning of our "athlete" adventure, Danny forgot to give himself his shot of long-acting insulin in the morning. I found it on his desk before dinner that night and finally understood why he'd had high numbers all day. I called the nurse diabetes educator and asked her what to do.

She suggested giving him half his normal dose of long-acting insulin immediately, giving him a larger than normal dose in the morning, then resuming our regular pattern the next day. She said his numbers would probably go high or low as a result, but it was the best we could do. I didn't like the idea of giving him too little insulin and then too much.

I was aware of not wanting to offend her. I took a deep breath and asked, "What would happen if we just kept his numbers down tonight with short-acting insulin and started him on his regular dose tomorrow?"

"Well, you could do that, but it would mean you'd have to get up with him every three hours at night," she said. It struck me then that even though she'd been our primary nurse for a year, she didn't know us. We'd shown her our schedule, and it obviously hadn't registered that we always got up at night and would always choose the best route over the easiest one.

I asked her which would be in his best interest, and she said, "Well, the short-acting would be much better." It scared me to think that if I hadn't suggested this option, she wouldn't have mentioned it. I reported that we'd reduced Danny's carbs after four o'clock in the afternoon and told her how much better his nighttime numbers were. All she said was, "Oh." No curiosity, no congratulations, no connection. I couldn't help but add, "I wish someone had told me this two years ago." She told me to call if I had any more questions. I couldn't think of anything more to say. Our relationship was a benign one, but it was finally clear that this medical team didn't appreciate what we were doing any more than the last one.

I refused to accept that this was the best we could do.

Brian and I had a conversation about how both our diabetes medical teams appeared to see everyone who came to them as unwilling to extend himself or herself, and as a result, taught to the lowest common denominator. They didn't want to offend parents and they didn't want to create stress, both worthy goals, but they were also so blinded by their low expectations that when they encountered a family that was willing to push itself, they didn't rise to the occasion. We didn't want to settle, and so we began yet another search.

A Like-Minded Diabetes Team, Finally

Barry Sears wrote *The Zone Diet,* and one of his colleagues, Dr. Eric Freedland, lives in my town, doing research on the effects of nutrition on diabetes. I'd often read his column on one of my favorite Web sites, diabetesincontrol.com, and so I picked up the phone and called him.

I explained what we were trying to do in a few sentences, and Dr. Freedland responded with excitement and enthusiasm. "That's it," he said. "This is the cutting edge of what we're finding right now. Regulating the quality of the carbohydrates and limiting their amount is so important." He launched into his fears about where the current trend, "a carb is a carb," was leading us. He and his colleagues were finding that some children with Type 1 diabetes were eating so poorly that they were becoming insulin-resistant and developing Type 2 diabetes as well.

"High-carbohydrate diets stress an already stressed system."

I asked him to explain.

"High-glycemic foods like candy and white bread have been proven to raise inflammatory markers in the body. It's complicated to explain why, but you don't want those markers to be high." I couldn't believe I'd found a person who could give me scientific reasons for why we'd been avoiding spaghetti and baked potatoes.

We met for coffee and talked for hours. He knew a lot of the researchers and nutritional experts who'd influenced my thinking. We formed an instant rapport, and our conversation was like a game of tennis, volleying facts, research, and books across the net. A doctor and I were playing the same game for once, and it was so much fun I couldn't stop smiling. He said he'd do his best to find someone to work with us.

The next day, Dr. Freedland referred me to Jan Hangen, a nutritionist at Children's Hospital Boston who believed in low-carbohydrate, high-fiber, whole foods diets for children with both Type 1 and Type 2 diabetes. She worked with an endocrinologist, Dr. Maryanne Quinn, and a diabetes nurse educator, Kristen Rice, and Dr. Freedland felt they'd be a good support for a family like ours.

I called the doctor he'd recommended immediately. Even though she worked at Children's Hospital, Dr. Maryanne Quinn answered her own phone! I told her why I was calling, and she said she thought our diet sounded great and agreed that a Hemoglobin A1c of 7.8 was too high for our efforts. After urging me to contact Jan, the nutritionist, she connected me to the switchboard so I could make an appointment.

Jan was equally lovely. We'd read the same authors and we ate the same way. I asked if she could teach me why Danny's blood sugars were so variable when he ate so well and we monitored him so closely. She said, "Don't worry. Just come on in and I'll teach you all I know." I called Brian to tell him I thought I'd finally found the team we'd been looking for.

That night my sister, Julie, helped me draft this letter to our previous team:

Dear Dr. J,

Brian and I wanted to let you know that we have decided to change to another medical team. In telling you this, we also wanted to explain what has fueled our decision in the genuine hope that it may change how you meet the challenge of working with families like us in the future.

When Danny was first diagnosed, our only objective was to learn how to keep Danny safe and alive with exogenous insulin. Our original medical team was wonderful at helping us manage those frantic first months, but as we researched and networked, we began to realize that many lifestyle issues, such as exercise, nutrition and complementary or alternative medicine, were not being addressed. We noticed that Danny's body responded very differently to low-glycemic index/high-fiber foods. He also responded very well to acupuncture. We came to you because your hospital was recommended as a "progressive" setting where we could do more for Danny than simply giving him insulin.

In our first meeting with your nutritionist, we were shocked to find that for a disease that requires a food diary, there was no education or discussion about the quality of the food. Outside of endocrinology, it is hard to find anyone who believes that a carb is a carb anymore. We worry that diabetes educators are missing a huge opportunity to educate parents about making better food choices. I think the fear of putting pressure on parents leads diabetes educators to avoid saying that a breakfast of fruit with whole grain bread is better for kids with diabetes than Fruit Loops.

Brian and I, like many parents, are very committed and want to know the *best* way, not necessarily the easiest way, to help Danny continue to be happy and healthy. We have not been satisfied with Danny's latest Hemoglobin A1c results of 8.1 and 7.8 so we decided on our own that our family would sharply reduce carbohydrates after Danny's four o'clock snack.

Danny was happy to go along because we were all eating the same foods. His two-week average is now 140 instead of 180.

Last week I found a nutritionist who was excited about our diet. She believes, as we do, that diabetes is not just about the pancreas and insulin, but requires support for the child's whole system. When she said, "I can provide you with all kinds of information," I realized that this kind of enthusiasm and openness is what we have been seeking.

The doctor who works with Jan assured me that she teaches about the benefits of healthy eating and says she will work with us to ensure consistently better numbers for Danny. We are going to move to their practice in the hope that their approach will not only lead to improvement in Danny's numbers, but support healthier lifestyle choices for our whole family.

Sincerely,

Laura Plunkett

I received a very nice reply. Dr. J was glad we'd found what we were looking for and said that we'd always be welcome back to her practice.

CHAPTER 8

Our Family at Two Years

Our Second Christmas

Last year we'd ordered Chinese food on Christmas Eve and eaten it with Brian's brother Conor and his family before going to a church wassail party preceding the religious service. The unlimited access Danny had to desserts and apple cider at the party meant we were up all night, giving him shots to lower his blood sugar levels. He was miserable because he still hadn't been able to eat all the things he wanted. We were miserable because we hated saying "no" to Danny, especially on Christmas Eve.

The next day I served a full Christmas dinner for our entire extended family, and our guests brought delicious desserts, which Danny sampled. After Brian and I cooked, cleaned, served, and paid attention to Danny's numbers all day, Danny's blood sugars weren't in the target range once. I burst into tears and told Brian I never wanted to have Christmas at our house again.

A year later, I was determined to do it differently. We invited both of Brian's brothers and their families for Christmas Eve dinner, but I talked with everyone ahead of time. When I explained how hard it was for us to prepare the food as well as take care of Danny, my sister-in-law Erica offered to make steak tips and salad at our house. Brian's brother Duffy brought mashed potatoes and green beans. Then Danny and Brian played floor hockey in the basement while everyone else went to the wassail party. Danny's blood sugar was actually low from exercise when he arrived at church for the service.

The first thing Danny said was, "I really wish I could have a cookie," and I was able to say, "Take any one you want," with a light heart. He said, with a big smile, "I'll get a small one so I don't spike."

On Christmas Day, we served a big turkey dinner, and everyone helped. Conor washed most of the dishes, Erica cleaned up, and the only dessert was my mother-in-law's low-sugar cheesecake. Danny had a small slice with lots of strawberries, and he was happy. That night I felt like we had navigated our way through this holiday more successfully. We were exhausted, but content.

A Change in Perspective

After a month of our no-carbs-after-four o'clock plan, Danny was on eight units of long-acting Lantus, 30 percent less than he'd been getting, and we'd cut his Novolog in half. After Christmas, his numbers started to rise again. It was impossible to know whether it was the excitement of Christmas, a growth spurt and hormonal changes, or our loosened vacation routine. It could have been the fact that Danny had missed two weeks of reflexology or perhaps something that hadn't occurred to us. His need for insulin was on an upward spiral again.

It still threw me for a loop every time the progress we were so excited about evaporated and disappeared. Life at home was so tense that, one evening, Brian and I put Danny to bed, left Jessie in charge, and went out to a local bar to have a drink. It had been an endless day with the kids bickering over everything and Danny's numbers still in the two and three hundreds, though we tested him every two hours and gave him shots with every meal and snack. No matter how much he ate, he kept complaining he was starving. We both desperately needed an attitude adjustment.

The bar was crowded, and a basketball game was on the television when we arrived. People were talking about the latest trades in the NBA and which beer to order. Some were actually laughing. Somehow, I'd forgotten how light and relaxed the rest of the world could be and how much we needed to get out once in a while.

Brian and I took a seat, ordered drinks, and made sure our cell phones had service. We promised each other we wouldn't mention diabetes or the kids. The bartender filled us in on the game, and for a few minutes we sat glued to the television. My White Russian was sweet and strong, the bar was loud, and the room was dark. No one needed anything. I felt small, just one of sixty people in the room. One of millions in the world. And all of us were only human, just trying to get through life one step at a time. Slowly I started to feel a new perspective creeping over me.

I gave Brian a poke and yelled in his ear, "We can handle this. We'll just raise his insulin some more and keep going. Life could be a lot worse."

He smiled, looking more relaxed than he had all day. "I know," he said. "It gets so damn tense. We have to remember we can only do what we can do."

Even though we were tempted, we limited ourselves to one drink each. We knew there were special dangers to drinking to excess, including that we might sleep through the alarm and find in the morning that something had happened to Danny. After an hour, we headed home arm-in-arm.

Jessie was watching a movie, but we talked her into playing a board game with us in the family room. Our mood was contagious, and even she was cheered up by the end. We tried to explain that we'd been so tense because we'd forgotten that being happy actually helped us function better, and that enjoying life was as high a priority as getting everything right. As I tucked her in that night, I hoped that once we were back in our usual school routine, we could remember to hold on to that feeling.

The Elements of Wonderful Medical Care

Our meeting with Dr. Quinn was a pilgrimage. Brian, Jessie, Danny, my cousin Sarah, who's slightly older than Jessie, and I all showed up. Dr. Quinn laughed when she saw our entourage filing into her office. We were looking forward to meeting her because she'd responded to our letter of introduction with friendly and thoughtful e-mails, a first for us. We weren't disappointed. She was funny, warm, and intelligent. The girls perched on her examining table, and we all listened with rapt attention as she told us that she herself had had diabetes since she was four years old, and that she was currently on a low-carbohydrate, low-glycemic index diet herself. She even asked for the recipe of my organic nut cookies and joked that maybe we should write a cookbook together.

Dr. Quinn emphatically recommended the pump, which she used herself. She felt that it would enable us to get better results, but she didn't want to force it on Danny. He wasn't eager to try it because, he said, "I like the way we do it now." She suggested he read about it on some Web sites.

Though none of our other doctors had valued it, Dr. Quinn praised us for helping Danny have such a long honeymoon. When we told her that we were disappointed that healthy nutrition wasn't stressed in diabetes education, she explained that sometimes members of a diabetes team don't want to put too heavy a burden on distressed parents and that only twenty percent of her patients were as motivated as we were. Dr. Quinn was the first doctor who actually seemed to accept and trust our way of doing things. She said to us, "I can tell how hard you're trying," and "I can see how committed you are."

She complimented us by saying, "Wow, eating this way is a huge commitment," and telling Jessie, "What a good sister you are to do this with Danny."

When I mentioned that I had given up working, she surprised me by looking me in the eye and asking what I used to do. We all felt heard and respected. It was a remarkable meeting.

Following that appointment, Danny's numbers became even less predictable. The next day, mid-afternoon, Danny was 327. We gave him five units of Novolog and two hours later, he was 33, close to the danger zone. How could it be that sometimes five units were too much and sometimes weren't nearly enough? It drove us crazy not to know.

I'd cautiously mentioned giving Danny a C-peptide test to see if he was still producing his own insulin, a possible explanation for Danny's unpredictable swings, and Dr. Quinn had ordered one. We found out he was only producing trace amounts of insulin. After twenty-four months, the honeymoon was officially over. It was better to know.

We were incredibly tired when we entered Jan Hangen's office a week later. She met us with a huge smile, said she'd had a long conversation with Dr. Quinn, and was "excited to meet with the whole Plunkett clan." Her casual friendliness shocked all four of us out of our lethargy.

Our previous nutritionists had always entered the components of Danny's meal plan into a computer to obtain the fat, protein, and carbohydrate contents. Since his meals were usually within the desirable range, they'd then tell us we were doing a good job, though his carbohydrates were on the low side, and remind us of the importance of serving him his favorite foods.

Jan, on the other hand, asked about our typical breakfasts of organic yogurt, homemade granola and blueberries, or a fruit shake, and said, "Obviously, these are much better choices than you could be making, but let's see if we can improve them." She wanted us to give Danny *fewer* carbohydrates at breakfast and extolled the virtues of eggs, which Danny wouldn't touch. This set off a long conversation between Jan and Danny about the importance of protein and the right type of fats. She pushed salmon, eggs, and chicken, and tried to convince him to give up butter, cheese, and bacon.

It was not one of Danny's favorite conversations. Jessie started squirming the moment she realized Jan was trying to convince us to make even more changes to our diet. Brian protested that he absolutely could not give up butter. In response, she launched into the virtues of olive oil, walnut oil, avocado, and almonds as fat sources. I was stunned, amazed that someone else was taking charge. Jan had opinions and suggestions and she knew much more than I did. She was talking about things I cared about. I was on the edge of my seat and hungry for information. I swear my whole body tingled with relief.

I'd found a source of raw milk, and I mentioned to Jan that I'd heard that raw milk was carefully regulated for bacteria now. I was prepared for her to warn us against it. Instead, her eyes lit up and she raved about the enzymes in the milk, its high-fat content, which counteracts its carbohydrates, and raw milk's low-glycemic index compared to pasteurized milk. She considered it a highly nutritious option.

When Jan looked at our food log, she pointed out ways we could improve. She emphasized that every time Danny had carbohydrates, he should also have protein and good fats to avoid spikes. She instructed us to make sure he got both soluble and insoluble fibers, as well as cooked and uncooked vegetables.

When she heard about our blood sugar troubles after the holidays, Jan wondered why we hadn't called Dr. Quinn. She assured us that both of them wanted us to keep in close touch. She also said that Dr. Quinn wanted to meet with Brian and me alone in a month, so that we'd have time to talk. Having seen our former doctors every six months, we were astonished.

After we left Jan's office, Brian gave me a hug. He was proud of me for sticking with my convictions. The kids, on the other hand, were sullen, and once we reached the car, they started to complain. Danny reminded us that he hated fish and eggs and would never like them. Jessie said Jan was too bossy and, in her opinion, we'd already made enough changes.

Now that we'd finally found what we'd been looking for, I should have felt elated and strong, but as the kids argued and shoved each other, I realized that I was at the end of my resources again. Finding a way to make eggs look tempting to Danny seemed to call for super-heroic powers while all I wanted was to put cold cereal on the table or call out for pizza. I leaned back in the car seat and said nothing.

When the kids went back to school, however, I started to sort myself out. We added a handful of almonds, a cheese stick, or a slice of deli meat to the popcorn, apple sauce, or carrot sticks in Danny's lunchbox. I started using olive oil in place of butter. I reassured Danny that we weren't going to force a salmon omelet on him, but that we expected him to try fish and eggs when we ate them. I started talking to Danny about the pros and cons of the pump.

At last, I could see a pattern emerging. My spirit would hit bottom, and I'd give in to the feeling that I couldn't do or change one more thing. Then time would pass until one morning I woke to find I had gotten my second wind. It was reassuring.

Brian had had a tough time too. After feeling we were solidly on the right road in December, we saw Danny's insulin needs rise after the holidays. What wore Brian down was that the ratio of insulin to carbohydrates, how much insulin Danny needed to handle a certain number of grams, always seemed to be changing. Also, we couldn't predict the amount one unit of insulin would lower his blood sugar level.

"It's terribly frustrating," he said to me one night. "With no precise formula, you never have any reason for confidence. It's one thing if you're dropping the ball, but when you're doing everything you can and the results are still so variable, it's irritating and disappointing.

"Our new doctor is much warmer than our others and because she has diabetes herself, she really seems to understand. She thought our numbers at our first appointment were good, but that was then. Now he's having wide swings between highs and lows and after all this time, it's discouraging."

Brian and I both had those feelings, but we tried to protect Danny from them. He wanted us to be in control so that he could be a kid and go about his life. My father kept suggesting that we hand over more responsibility to Danny, but if we couldn't manage it, how was he supposed to?

At this point Dr. Quinn called with good news. She had Danny's Hemoglobin A1c for October, November, and December, and it was 6.8, which was the lowest it had been. Even though getting excited over numbers was emotional suicide, I was excited anyway since my understanding was that staying under seven significantly reduced the likelihood of long-term complications. That number covered the time Danny had spent with so few carbohydrates in the evening and in my heart, I knew that had made the difference. Now that we had done it once, I thought we could do it again.

Even over the phone, I could feel how much Dr. Quinn cared, and I realized she was offering to become another support for us. She didn't rush as she asked questions and we began formulating a new treatment plan. She suggested more Lantus, less Novolog, and a carbohydrate to insulin ratio of seven grams to one unit, instead of ten to one as we'd been doing. She actually explained how she and Jan had figured this out and told me to call her in a few days to let them know how it was working. No doctor had ever asked for a follow-up call before.

Kristen Rice, the team's diabetes nurse educator, was the same way. She was funny, smart, and down-to-earth. She laughed from deep in her belly and seemed to have all the time in the world for our questions. In fact, when I offered to e-mail the numbers on Danny's log to her, she said she preferred phone calls because then we could spend more time working on strategies together. When I thought of the team Dr. Quinn had assembled, I had a catch in my throat. I'd never know as much as they did or have to worry that they'd spare us the hard work involved.

From the beginning, I'd had a vision of the four people in our family as four legs under a table, all of us needing to be strong and sturdy to avoid disaster. As I got off the phone with Dr. Quinn, I had the feeling that with three more legs under our table, we were solid now.

A Successful Weekend Away

In January 2004, Brian and I took two nights and three days away without the kids. We were sooo happy! No emergencies and no panic. Every time we called to check, everyone was having a good time.

The scheduling was a bit complicated. On Saturday night, Danny stayed with his best friend, Zach, whose mother, Robin, was confident that she could handle anything that came up. Jessie stayed with my sister, Julie, and her two younger cousins. On Sunday night, after dinner, my parents picked up both kids and put them to bed at their house. On Monday, which was Martin Luther King Day, Jessie, Danny, and my mom went to the Museum of Science first thing in the morning. Jessie took a computer course from nine to five while Danny and my mom hung out at the museum for eight hours straight.

My mother packed two snacks and followed my instructions about what Danny liked to eat at the museum cafeteria, so lunch and dinner went smoothly. They saw an Omnimax movie about tigers, went to a show about the *Titanic*, observed a program on electricity, visited the gift shop, dipped into a few exhibits, and hung out in the computer room. Danny performed his own blood tests, figured out his own doses, and gave himself shots in the stomach. My mother kept track of the clock. His blood sugars stayed within limits, and there were *no* mishaps.

That night my mother dropped Jessie and Danny off with these final words, "Well, Laura, you've been wishing for a miracle. Maybe this is it."

Danny's Advice

When Brian and I got back, we decided we wanted to invite two families for Friday night dinner before we all went to watch the town's biggest January event, a bonfire of discarded Christmas trees. For the life of me, I couldn't figure out an easy and inexpensive way to feed ten people a low-carbohydrate meal. When I asked Jessie and Danny, both of them wistfully came up with the idea of having real honest-to-goodness House of Pizza pizza. I talked to Danny as he was getting ready for bed Thursday night, feeling guilty about putting him on the spot.

"Danny," I said," we're having the Traynors and the Rileys over for dinner tomorrow night before the bonfire and I can't figure out a fast, low-carbohydrate way to feed them. I was wondering how you'd feel if we ordered pizza for everyone else and got you something different."

"That's okay," he said immediately, "as long as I can have a chicken Caesar salad."

The next day, I bought Danny pizza for lunch. That night he explained to everyone that he'd already had pizza and then happily ate his salad. He didn't mind testing, he didn't mind shots, and now he didn't mind watching people eat his favorite food in front of him.

Later that night, as I tucked Danny into bed, I asked him what he could remember about the time his blood sugar ran low on his first trip to the Museum of Science with his grandmother. He gave me an uncomprehending look. He couldn't remember the event even when I described what had happened. We talked about how long ago that had been and how many things had changed since then.

"What would you say to a seven-year-old boy who'd just found out he had diabetes?" I asked.

"I'd tell him that it will all get better in the end," he said. "My life is a lot better now than right after I found out. I'm used to eating this way and now I like the taste of things I didn't used to. The new insulin, like Lantus, and the new meters keep making things easier and I'm getting better at dealing with everything, like it's easier to know when you're low when you've had diabetes longer, even though sometimes when I feel low, I'm high.

"Also, I'd tell him to test at halftime if he plays soccer. After soccer and mountain biking, I always get an exercise high. Dad says that's because it's vigorous.

"That's all. It just gets better."

Jessie's Reflections

A couple of nights later, Jessie and I sat on her bed and talked about the changes we had been through. "Now that I'm thirteen, I realize that I know a lot about diabetes," she said. "I still think about when we first went to the hospital. When I look back, the classes at the hospital were a lot like the Game of Life. You know how in that board game, there's a choice between going to college and choosing life experience? One day you took me out of school and let me learn about life.

"Lots of things are better than they were at first. Everyone is much more relaxed. Danny's remembering to test and take shots. He tells us when he's feeling low and doesn't cry or whine half as much. Our diet is better, and even if I had the opportunity to go back to before Danny had diabetes, I wouldn't. We're all closer since we've been through these hard times together."

Then she added, "All we can do now is hope for a cure."

Brian's Philosophy

Meanwhile, Brian was completely used to our schedule. He woke up at six, went downstairs, made yogurt with blueberries and granola, or some kind of fruit shake for Danny, and gave him his multivitamins. If Jessie was up, Brian fed her too and helped make her lunch. He unloaded the dishwasher, made Danny's lunch as well as two snacks, and checked the diabetes supplies for school. I came downstairs by six thirty to help, and then I would take over while Brian showered and got ready for work. We were all out the door by seven thirty.

During the day, Brian called home just to touch base. We didn't get a lot of private time at home, so we did some of our best talking on the phone. Brian tried to leave work around five thirty, which got him home by train at about six thirty. He would eat the dinner I made, then help with homework or exercise with the kids. He usually read to Danny and Jessie, and then we'd try to find time to connect.

Danny always tested himself before bed and then, depending upon the numbers, Brian would set the alarm to wake up between one and three o'clock to test Danny again. About half the time, he didn't have to do anything, but Brian gave Danny milk if he was low and insulin if he was high. Many mornings Brian was groggy, and his caffeine intake definitely increased. Having a rhythm in the mornings really helped, however, because no matter how tired he was, he knew exactly what had to be done and how long it would take. Our morning routine made the whole day go better, and Brian slept as late as he wanted on the weekends because I always got up with Danny.

Some men, I guess, might have resented having to do so much at home, but Brian had an acceptance of our new reality that was characteristic of his personality in general. "I believe we each have our own path to lead," he told me. "Mine is to support my family and try to be as happy as possible."

Even before Danny got ill, Brian made conscious choices about how much of his life would be claimed by his work. Back in law school, he began defining success as having the freedom to make choices that gave him satisfaction. The result was that his present law firm was his sixth as a commercial finance attorney. Searching for the right place, he intentionally sought out people of high character and strong family orientation who valued having a certain amount of time to devote to other things. Of course, he wanted to make as much money as possible, but only if he could achieve a successful balance between work and the rest of his life.

In many law firms, lawyers are "service partners." They operate at a partner level, but the clients are not theirs, which means that they're dependent on another lawyer to generate the work they do. They not only have to keep clients satisfied, they have to make the "rainmaking" partner happy as well. If the senior partner's goal is to make as much money as possible, he works the service partner as hard as he can. Therefore, as soon as he could, Brian focused on finding his own clients. He knew it would be a lot easier to create the life he wanted when he generated business himself and made his own decisions.

"Thinking about how much has changed since Danny's illness, I've come to see that life is a lot like a wave machine which is constantly in motion," he said to me, explaining his philosophy of life. "Every one of us is on a surfboard and sometimes you're going up the wave, sometimes you're riding the wave, and sometimes you wipe out. The machine takes no notice and just keeps going, like life, so if you fall off, you have no choice but to get back on your board and try to find a new equilibrium.

"Although it's possible to achieve balance over a lifetime, it may not be particularly satisfying at any one particular time," he acknowledged. "Sometimes you're doing a little of everything and not enough of anything. If you're stuck on one wave for a long time, some part of you inevitably ends up being unfulfilled. But, if you acknowledge that it's only for a while, you know that's just where you are at the moment."

Of course, Brian's continually altering his view of the moment. "A moment can be a day, a week, a year, or longer," he said. "I take the long view and look at this as a ten-year moment before Danny grows up and becomes fully responsible for managing his own diabetes. When my family obligations lessen, then I'll reconsider how I spend my time."

For example, his jujitsu practice now takes a back seat to Danny's needs. After college, Brian was training three or four times a week. When he became a lawyer with a wife and children, he felt lucky to get to the dojo once a week. Right after Danny's diagnosis, he gave it up completely, but now he's back to once a week, which he sees as both good and bad. It's good because he's still doing jujitsu while many of his contemporaries have disappeared from the dojo, and his skills continue to increase. It's bad because he doesn't get to train as much as he'd like to, and he's not improving at the same rate he did when he was younger.

"I can either be unhappy that I'm no longer at my earlier level or be thrilled that at age forty-one, I've just earned my third-degree black belt," he explained. "When I measure my progress from the perspective of my whole life, I choose to be thrilled." He was even able to get away last summer for an overnight jujitsu seminar in New Hampshire. It wasn't the three- or four-day camp he used to go to, but it was still fun.

"I don't know why Danny has diabetes," he concluded, summing up. "I didn't cause it, he didn't cause it, and this is just the path our lives will take from here on. Life could be better, but it could also be a lot worse. I've seen how involved your parents are with their children and grandchildren, and it's made me realize that family obligations never end; they simply change as your family grows. That's the way I think it should be. To me that's a successful family."

Brian isn't filled with regret about Danny's diabetes. "What would the regret be?" he asked me. "That I chose to have children? I have more fun with my kids than most parents do, I think, because I love to play. Parenting isn't easy, and we've given up so much of our independence in the past few years, but Danny and Jessie give our lives meaning."

Danny's Final Word on the Subject

Brian and Danny were at the Food Court at the Mall.

"Dad, when someone gets three wishes from the genie in the lamp, why don't they just wish for more wishes?" Danny asked.

"Well, if you had three wishes, what would you wish for?"

"I don't know. I pretty much have everything I want."

"Well, the first thing I'd wish for is that you didn't have diabetes anymore."

"Diabetes isn't so bad. It hasn't changed things that much." Danny looks down at the chicken and veggies on his plate and brightens. "Look, it's got us eating healthier food. Otherwise, I'd be eating French fries!"

CHAPTER 9

▼

Postscript at Three and One-Half Years (A1c 6.2)

The Pump

Our transition to the pump in the third year of Danny's illness transformed the rhythms of our family in so many ways that it's hard to explain why we waited so long. I can only say that attaching a machine to your child's body twenty-four hours a day seemed like an extreme step to take when you are still struggling to make everything feel normal. That's why, when toward the end of the second year, Dr. Quinn strongly suggested to Danny that he consider the pump, we didn't apply pressure. Everyone agreed that a child needed to be ready or the transition to the pump wouldn't work.

Dr. Quinn, however, was convinced we would appreciate the flexibility the pump offered and gain better blood glucose control, so Danny and I took a few baby steps to familiarize ourselves with it. First, we visited the secretary at our church who'd had diabetes since she was a teenager. She showed us how the pump connected to her body and demonstrated how she could turn up the insulin while she was sitting at her desk and reduce it while she was exercising. When she explained that she could eat whatever and whenever she wanted, Danny was intrigued. He thought the pump, which resembled a pager or a beeper, looked "cool."

Second, Danny and I looked at different brands on the Internet. Each Web site taught about the pump through video games, and since Danny didn't get a lot of computer time, he was happy to spend some time playing. However, he still didn't want to try one.

Finally, in front of Danny, I talked to Brian about what I'd learned.

"Did you know that the only time you get a shot is when you change the site every two or three days?" or "Did you know that if we had to give Danny insulin at night, we could push a button instead of waking him up?" or "I can't believe that if Danny wanted to eat every ten minutes, he'd just log small amounts of carbohydrates into the pump and it would do the rest. He wouldn't have to eat his food all at one time anymore." During this phase, Danny announced that he wanted the pump.

Our medical team needed to be sure that he was clearly interested before they would okay the prescription. Danny met with our nurse educator and confided that his biggest and only fear was inserting the needle. It was long and thick. Wouldn't it hurt? Kristen was very honest with him. Yes, it probably would, but not as much as he imagined. She took out a sample infusion set and showed him both the mechanical inserter and how one did it manually. We all held our breath as Danny pinched a roll of his belly and slowly slid the long needle into his stomach by hand. Jessie and I fought the urge to look away while Brian and Kristen leaned in and watched. It was over before we knew it.

"It hurt a little, but it's no big deal," Danny commented.

I'd read that the transition to the pump sometimes went better when a parent wore one as well, so I ordered "a loaner" and it arrived with Danny's permanent one. A week later, a pump representative came to our house to teach us how to use it. Our family assembled in the living room, and Danny and I programmed our pumps together. We'd have saline in both pumps for one week. Then, when we next met with Kristen at the hospital, Danny would change to insulin.

Danny inserted his site first. Too soon, it was my turn. I took a deep breath and slowly pushed the needle in. How bad could it be? He hadn't even flinched. Actually, the pain of insertion completely stunned me. I faked a smile and pushed it in all the way, still holding my breath. Everyone clapped and I exhaled. Thank goodness I wouldn't have to do it again for two more days.

I had the opportunity to experience what Danny now took for granted. I learned to enter the carbohydrate value for every bite of food I ate. I changed the "temporary basal rate" when I exercised or watched a movie. When I changed my clothes, I clipped the pump to my underwear or disconnected it, and when I showered, I capped the site to protect it. I learned to sleep with a hard plastic rectangle attached to my body and to make sure the tubing didn't get tangled or catch on anything. The two days flew by.

Then it was time for both of us to change the sites. I filled the reservoirs with saline and primed the tubing, so that the only thing left was to connect the two pumps to ourselves. "Danny," I called cheerfully from our family room, "time to change our sites."

Danny had friends coming soon, so he went first, quickly stripping away the packaging, swabbing a new place on his belly and sliding the needle in with a quiet "Ow!" He clipped his pump to his jeans, pulled his shirt down and went to see if his friends had come.

"Hey, what about me?" I called, and Jessie yelled in from the kitchen, "Don't worry, Mom, I'm here as long as I don't have to watch." Alone, I had no one to be brave for. I took the needle, pierced my skin, and got about halfway. This was no joke. It hurt, my hand was shaking, and all I could think about was that Danny would have to do this a million times. I couldn't make myself push the needle any further.

Danny came back in. "No one's here yet. How's it going?" He looked down at my stomach. "Mom, you have to put it all the way in."

"I know," I replied, "I'm taking a break."

He straightened up and looked at me. "I already know how to do it. You don't have to." Jessie joined him. "Why are you doing that? Danny can do it himself." As I pulled the needle out, I tried to give the impression that they'd had to convince me. In the end, although I did learn how to program and use the pump, I never mastered site insertion.

More importantly, Danny did.

When we met with Kristen again a week later, we filled Danny's pump reservoir with insulin and were off and running. That was the beginning of a newfound sense of freedom. All of a sudden it didn't matter how much or how often Danny ate. He could eat an apple at 3:00 PM, a glass of milk at 3:20 PM, and a bag of popcorn at 3:30 PM. All he had to do was enter carbohydrate and blood sugar numbers, and the pump did the calculations for him: no shots, no complicated math, no time constraints. In addition, if Danny wasn't hungry, he didn't have to eat.

Now, if Danny and Brian went biking, Danny could set up a steady dose of insulin at a reduced rate, and he didn't have to stop to eat every five minutes. If Danny wanted to watch a movie, he could increase his insulin supply and lie on the couch without going high. He could detach the pump for soccer games or to swim for an hour, then reattach it briefly to give himself whatever dose he needed. As one mother put it on kidsrpumping.com, "The insulin pump is not the cure and it's not without frustrations, but it is *liberating*!"

Our pump experience hasn't been perfect. There have been times when the injection site dislodged or the tubing got kinked, and we didn't notice until Danny's high numbers indicated a problem. He has red bumps on his belly where the old sites haven't healed yet, which are more noticeable than injection spots. He once went water skiing at camp and forgot to remove his pump; it was only luck that it was there at the end of the afternoon. Even with the pump, Danny continues to have some highs and lows during the night so we continue to check him if he is out of range before bed. He still needs exercise after eating a big meal.

Yet his numbers are so improved, and Danny's life is so much easier and more spontaneous, that we cannot imagine life without the pump. Three months after he started the pump, Danny's Hemoglobin A1c number was 6.2, its lowest level. Three and six months later, it was 6.3. The pump not only gave us more freedom, it clearly gave us better control. Now Danny wouldn't think of going back to shots.

One seductive aspect to the pump, however, is that it allows children to eat more of the typical American diet. Because the pump is so efficient, it's easier to get relatively good blood sugar numbers while eating sweets, fried foods, and high-carbohydrate meals. While we're grateful that Danny can now have a slice of pizza and ice cream at a party without automatically raising his numbers, we still limit these foods. I am totally convinced that a child with diabetes needs to keep his body as healthy as possible.

Laura: If I Only Knew Then What I Know Now

Though I don't claim we've become experts in raising a child with diabetes, we've certainly gotten wiser over time. Things start to feel familiar: an extremely high or low blood sugar number, a missed dose of insulin, an emergency room visit, a string of broken nights' sleep, or the realization that the emergency kit is still at home. I've learned to comfort myself by saying, "I've handled this before. We can do this." The situations that made me cry in the beginning have gotten much easier. I got used to giving shots, to blood tests, to the limitations of my life. Tears don't rush to my eyes as I go through daily procedures, and I have become less sensitive as the brand-new has become well-known.

I've gotten better at taking things one step at a time and completely ignoring the big picture. Any situation is manageable if you concentrate on doing it for a week or a month. In a positive way, the future has become very indistinct. When I look at this week's numbers and hear myself thinking, "*What is this doing to his circulation, his kidneys, and his heart?"* I close the curtain in my mind and remember that I have no idea what the future holds. When I'm scared, I remind myself to look at Danny. What I see is that he's doing fine.

I have seen that diet has a *huge* effect on blood sugars and overall feelings of well-being. Although the transition was tough, once we were eating a more complex and reduced carbohydrate diet, we all felt better. Our taste buds expanded, and we all started liking more healthy foods. The results for Danny were a stronger immune system, fewer mood swings, an enhanced sense of well-being, more energy, and smaller blood sugar fluctuations.

Repeatedly, we struggled against the belief that limiting your child's food choices can cause eating disorders. All I know is that it hasn't happened in our family. In fact, the opposite is true. Although both my children are still young and things could change in an instant, they're both maintaining healthy weights and seem to be relatively unconcerned about body image. I think it helped that in situations when Danny wanted diet soda or carb-free candy, I could honestly say, "I wouldn't put that in my body, Dan, so how could I, in good conscience, let you put it in yours?"

I think the biggest factor in not creating issues around eating was presenting the changes to the kids in a positive light, explaining our reasons, rather than blaming it on the diabetes or seeing it as a deprivation. I shared what I learned with the kids and explained that we were making changes so that we'd all be healthier. Even if they complained occasionally, they were in agreement with the plan. Danny went from tolerating iceberg lettuce, to enjoying romaine in Caesar salad after a year, to declaring himself a fan of red leaf lettuce just the other day. Of course, we made exceptions for special events. When it was important to Danny, he could choose what to eat without guilt, and Jessie had no restrictions on what she ate away from home.

I wish I'd had more confidence. Danny's first two medical teams came so highly recommended that I'd often leave an appointment with the feeling they must be right. What's wrong with me? Why can't I be satisfied? Now I know that my search was vital and I have advice to give: Pay attention to what your family requires. Never give up looking for what you need to stay engaged and motivated. Each family has its own style, and it's important to trust yourself and your instincts when you decide whether you're satisfied with your medical team or not.

I wish I'd been better at asking for help directly, especially because a family coping with diabetes looks fine, making it hard for people to understand that support is still needed. I often presented myself as "back to normal" because I judged myself for feeling overwhelmed. I still do. I tried not to tell too many people how hard a time we were having because I didn't want to seem too sad, too needy, too whiny, or, heaven forbid, sorry for myself. No one likes being in crisis all the time; no one wants to be a burden or a bore. I forgot that if you let people in and tell the truth, the good friendships just get better.

As time went on and I realized we were going to survive, I started to open up. I talked about more of the sordid details: about the bruises on Danny's belly and arms from the shots or the way it felt to stand in Danny's room with Brian at three in the morning, not knowing how much insulin to give. When someone casually asked how I was doing, I'd joke, "Well, for someone who hasn't slept through the night in a year…" or "Considering that I live in my kitchen…" I just got sick of saying "fine" and told the truth no matter what it was. I remember the jolt I gave someone by saying, "I felt like I'd won the lottery this morning because everyone was still alive." Because of my honesty, I think my friends understood that if I was less available, it wasn't because I didn't care about them.

Every day Danny's diabetes reminds me that I don't want to miss an opportunity to connect. Contrary to my fears, everyone stuck around, and although it sounds corny, I think diabetes blew my heart open. I love my friends now more than I ever have.

Finally, I wish I'd known from the beginning that my family would return to feeling okay again. The scares and the stress taught us that even if we occasionally let one another down, we could really count on each other. We're back to laughing at stupid things and having lively conversations at dinner. The kids are slimmer and healthier, and they take being active for granted. Brian and I feel older because of all the responsibility, but we're having fun again, at last. We know we can lean on each other in a way we never did before, and we have learned to appreciate carefree moments.

Life seems even more precious.

The four of us feel held by a wider community. Our family and friends pulled us through, and we can feel the safety net underneath us. Now, for the first time, we're aware that we have something to offer. We're sharing our experience with Danny because we want to help families who are starting out as bewildered and overwhelmed as we were.

When a child develops diabetes, it's as if a door opens into a new world and you have no choice but to pass through it and find your future happiness there. Without knowing what's ahead, you must put one foot in front of another without any compass more important than your own deepest convictions. Though you may be surrounded by conflicting advice and endless demands upon your time and energy, we hope this book will help you look for your own answers and trust yourself to build a life that is satisfying and meaningful on your own terms.

May it be so.

PART III

▼

A Survival Guide for Parents

Diabetes Preparation

- Place the following in a fanny pack:

  Blood glucose meter
  Test strips
  Lancets
  Spare battery for the meter
  Alcohol swabs
  Ketone strips
  Glucose tabs
  Glucose gel
  Glucagon kit
  Information sheet
  Granola bars
  Other snacks
  Supplies for injections or pump

- Check the contents of the fanny pack each night so that it contains everything you need in the morning.

- Make up an information sheet with the following:

  Your child's name and birth date
  Health insurance information (if available)
  Doctors' numbers
  Preferred emergency room
  Family and emergency contact telephone numbers
  Symptoms of high and low blood sugars
  Clear instructions on how to treat symptoms

- Post the information sheet by the primary telephone in your home

Sample Medical Information Sheet

Emergency numbers:

Insurance information:

Hospital telephone numbers with preferred emergency room:

Doctor and nurse telephone numbers for weekday/evening/weekends:

Parents work, home and cell phone numbers:

Trusted family, friend and neighbor numbers:

My child has juvenile diabetes and requires your watchful eye. S/he is insulin-dependent and (wears an insulin pump/takes injections of—give names of insulin used). My child must take glucose tabs with him/her everywhere s/he goes. Off school grounds s/he must have his/her test kit, tabs, gel, and snacks as well. The nurse must know where s/he is if s/he leaves the building. S/he is usually very good at detecting changes early and taking care of her/himself. Unless s/he is experiencing a serious low, please trust his/her judgment and follow his/her lead. (You can adjust all this to your child's ability level.)

If my child says s/he "feels low" or appears overly tired, whiny, or oppositional, s/he must test his/her blood sugar level with the test kit immediately. S/he needs to test a clean finger as opposed to an arm because it will give the most accurate reading. Please do not leave my child alone or unattended until s/he has checked her/his level and has treated any problem and recovered fully.

The target blood sugar levels fall between 80 and 140:

- If s/he is under 80, s/he should take 1 glucose tablet, < 70= 2 tablets, < 60= 3 tablets.

- If s/he appears unable to test him/herself, or you do not have a test kit available, give him/her several glucose tablets and test as soon as possible. *It takes ten minutes for glucose tablets to take full effect.*

- If s/he is unable to chew tablets, empty a tube of gel into his/her cheek lining and send someone else to get medical help.

- If s/he appears to be entering a coma or having a seizure, have someone call 9-1-1 and locate someone who can give him/her a shot of glucagon.

- If s/he is over 250 (sometimes high levels feel like low ones), please have him/her drink some water. This helps bring down the numbers. Have her/him check the site of the pump (if applicable) and check for ketones. If s/he is over 250 on his/her second reading, please call the nurse or her/his parents. Thank you.

- Choose a daily log that fits your desired record-keeping style and decide who will maintain it.

Sample Daily Log

Date											
Time:											
Reading:											
Amt. of insulin:											
Carbs:											
Exercise:											
Comments:											
Time:											
Reading:											
Amt. of insulin:											
Carbs:											
Exercise:											
Comments:											
Time:											
Reading:											
Amt. of insulin:											
Carbs:											
Exercise:											
Comments:											
Total carbohydrates per day: Total amounts of insulin per day:											

- Designate one place where the diabetes kit and log are *always* kept at home.

- Purchase a carbohydrate counter and a glycemic index, available at any bookstore. Put them where you can easily refer to them.

- Choose one shelf, drawer, or cabinet to keep all your diabetes supplies (except the refrigerated insulin), including a folder with your prescriptions and medical records so that your family is not seeing "diabetes stuff" everywhere.

- If possible, get a cell phone so that your child, the school, and any important caretakers can reach you. Some companies offer free cell phone 9-1-1 service if you cannot afford the full plan.

- The Visiting Nurses Association provides in-home visits and can help you educate neighbors, friends, and school officials.

- In emergencies, a call ahead to the emergency room can sometimes speed registration and allow the staff to prepare for your child's specific needs.

Getting Support

- Attend Juvenile Diabetes Research Foundation (JDRF) coffees, then offer to host one yourself so you can meet families that live nearby.

- Ask a family member, friend, or relative to attend as many medical appointments with you as possible. Take notes to review later.

- Try to make major decisions jointly with significant others. Children are more likely to comply with demands if the adults in their lives agree.

- Make sure you trust the members of your medical team. If your questions are not being answered, if a nutritionist is dismissive of your concerns, or if your child doesn't like her doctor, it's worth looking further. This is a long-term relationship.

- Securing help with errands, food preparation, cooking, or cleaning will leave you with more energy to cope with difficult situations as they arise. Try to find someone, even a teenager, who can come in a few hours a week to help. This is not self-indulgence.

- People may let you down because of inattention, busyness, ignorance, lack of focus, or poor judgment, but they rarely do it on purpose. Take the role of coach and try to figure out what went wrong. Work together to make sure it doesn't happen again.

- Teachers, doctors, babysitters, and friends will all have different styles, whether they baby, nag, push, or hover over your child. Realizing that everyone reacts differently to illness will help your child adjust to a wide variety of encounters.

- Spend an evening discussing the progress you've made with those intimately involved in your child's care. Look for hidden gains. For example: complicated activities which now seem simple, rejected foods which are now acceptable, ways in which family members have adjusted. Remember to express your heartfelt appreciation to each other.

- Seek a confidant who encourages curiosity, hopefulness, and thinking outside the box. Find an accepting listener who can ask open-ended questions like "What's happening? How do you feel about it? What can you do differently?" The opportunity to express withheld thoughts can bring relief to your spirits and help you regain the energy to deal with what is happening.

- If something goes wrong in public, do not hesitate to appeal for help. You can say, "My child has diabetes and she's not feeling well. Can someone help me?" In every crowd there is likely to be someone familiar with diabetes who will step forward.

Family Strategies

- Include your children in any decisions or life changes your family makes. Explaining "why" and seriously listening to objections makes it easier to solicit their cooperation.

- Do your best to convince your child with diabetes that both of you are on the same side in confronting this disease. Stress the idea that you are teammates with the same goals.

- Ask for your children's help in working out strategies for coping. Ask for suggestions.

- Talk about any change before you implement it. Allow time for children to get used to new ideas. Familiarity and information often ease a child's resistance.

- Try timed trials. For example, "Let's do this for two weeks and then we'll reconsider it."

- If something doesn't work, ask, "What else could we do to achieve the same results?"

- Children are often responsive to the explanations and exhortations of experts. Ask a nutritionist, visiting nurse, or someone with diabetes to talk with your child about issues in contention between you.

- Siblings have a right to their own ambivalent feelings. As long as they treat their siblings with respect, their complaints can be met with a sympathetic, "I know. It's hard."

- Draw the line between honesty, which you appreciate, and hurtful insults, which should be out-of-bounds within any family.

- When your child plays at a friend's home, send snacks in the diabetes kit, along with your medical information sheet, and a list of times to test. Be available by cell phone, if possible.

- Sharing child care with the parents of children with diabetes is optimal. You can meet them at local Juvenile Diabetes Research Foundation coffees.

- Make an effort to find your child's siblings a place where they can shine. Aim for small classes, dedicated adults, or a caring community of faith.

- Children with diabetes are in mourning for their lost freedom to eat whenever and whatever they want. Try to be understanding and reassuring, no matter how negative your child is at mealtimes. Offering sympathy and compassion is more nourishing than giving foods that don't have nutritional value.

- Accept that you may have a low energy level, be disorganized, or become flustered in emergencies. Gratefully allow others to make up for your limitations without reproaching yourself. The best possible distribution of tasks is to have everyone in your circle of support playing to his or her strengths.

- Exercise as a family. Riding bikes, taking walks, jogging, swimming, or shooting baskets have healthful effects for everyone.

- Talk with others about what you want to tell your child about the long-term effects of diabetes. Figure out what best suits your own child's personality. Some children will be motivated by knowing that their compliance can prevent serious illness later; other children may become so fearful that they despair.

- Take note of anniversaries: Celebrate your survival. Mourn your losses. Tell stories from the early days. Take turns reflecting upon what each one of you has learned by naming something you can do now that you never dreamed you ever would. Each anniversary can be a demonstration of your family's surprising capacity to deal with challenges.

- Although children have to learn to deal with the consequences of their actions, having unmanageable numbers has far too many serious, long-term medical complications for a young child to fully understand. It's the parent's role to attempt to prevent those consequences until a child is reasonably mature.

- As we struggle with our own eating impulses, we know how hard it is to deny ourselves without support and encouragement. Think of your family as an organization like Weight Watchers. Your job is to keep a close eye on your child's ups and downs, set limits, and cheer him on.

Emotional Perspectives

- The longer you offer loving guidance and support, the deeper the child will internalize the attitude needed to give himself excellent self-care as a teenager and young adult.

- Your attitude toward your child's illness will be reflected in her treatment of herself.

- Try to find a positive side to being the parent of a child with diabetes, even if it feels like a big stretch. Have you discovered inner resources? Are you more mindful of the blessings you have? Focusing upon your gains will lead you to become wise rather than bitter, accepting rather than resentful, and alive instead of numb.

- Often the only choice you have is between not-so-great alternatives. This is not your fault. You are not all-powerful. The reality is that as long as your child is in your care, you will have to make many unsatisfactory decisions.

- Diabetes is often unpredictable. Cause doesn't always equal effect. Sometimes, no matter what you do, blood sugars go crazy. Taking this in stride will get easier over time.

- When your child is ready for sleepovers or camp, plan as carefully as you can, check up as often as you need to, then take your courage in hand and let your child go.

- Don't let worry limit your family's range of activities any more than necessary. Recognize that you can proceed with activities in spite of your anxiety.

- It's important to be optimistic and go after what you want until you meet up with a solid "No." A camp may never have had a child with diabetes before, but you have nothing to lose by asking. An aunt may be known for her sweet tooth, but if you provide her with recipes, you may find a sympathetic ally.

- Share your ideas and impressions with your medical team even if they don't ask for them. Low expectations can dampen your efforts to create supportive situations.

- At times, a spike in your child's blood sugars will prevent her from doing something she cares about. Be sympathetic, but remember that the sooner your child accepts the inevitability of setbacks and sees herself as resilient, the more flexible she will become.

Self-Care

- In the first month after diagnosis, go through your calendar and cancel nonessential meetings and engagements. You will need your undivided attention for yourself and your family.

- This is a time to learn to accept help gracefully. Figure out what you need from others and ask for it with an open heart, accepting that people refuse for many reasons, not necessarily because they do not care.

- The feeling of being truly appreciated is usually a sufficient reward for the people who reach out and help you.

- When you find yourself inundated with advice, write it down. Put it aside until you feel ready to think about it.

- Follow your own timetable. Everyone takes a different amount of time to adjust to a new path in life. The vigilance this illness requires takes a tremendous amount of energy. Make sure *you* are ready before you resume your normal activities. Listen to your heart.

- When you feel crazy, anxious, stressed, or depressed, remember half the parents of children with newly-diagnosed diabetes are on the same roller coaster.

- The word "e-motion" means that feelings "move" through us. If you can express yourself in private by crying or screaming, a calmer emotion will replace the craziness you feel. Leave your child with a friend, a neighbor, a relative, or a babysitter, and go someplace you can be alone. You can return to your responsibilities later.

- A night out with a friend, a yoga class, a hot bath after your child is asleep, a long walk, or a jog can set the stage for a quick shift in perspective.

- Keeping a journal helps you judge your progress. A few phrases written on a page can sum up your more challenging moments. Looking back, earlier entries will demonstrate how far you have come.

- Allow yourself to be mothered. A good friend can be a wonderful mother if you let her know what you need, whether it's a cup of tea, a hot meal, or a hug.

Nutrition

- When you make changes in your family's diet, explain that it is for everyone's overall health, not just because of diabetes. Eating more vegetables, fruits, and whole grains while avoiding sugar, white flour, and processed foods is good for everyone.

- When you shop, concentrate on the outer edges of the store where you find fresh produce, meat, fish, whole grain breads, dairy, and frozen fruits and vegetables. Avoid the cookie, cracker, juice, candy, and soda aisles.

- In order to build maximum health, buy foods with good nutritional value. It seems simple now, but in the beginning I thought Cheezits and Goldfish were a staple. If you can, choose organic produce, eggs, and meat without antibiotics or hormones.

- When you get home, wash and cut up the vegetables and put them on a shelf in the refrigerator so that they are the first thing your children see when they open the door.

- While adjusting to a new diagnosis, do not bring your child with you to the supermarket because all the tempting things that spike blood sugars will be on full display.

- Do not have food in the house that a child with diabetes cannot eat. Encourage other family members to satisfy their sweet tooth away from home.

- Recommended cookbooks:
  Living on Live Foods by Alissa Cohen
  Nourishing Traditions by Sally Fallon with Mary Enig, Ph.D.
  Low-Carb Slow Cooker Recipes by *Better Homes and Gardens*

- When you know your child is going to be tempted by sweets away from home, send along a replacement treat, like sugar-free gum, to eat in place of candy.

- Feed your child at home before parties. This will help him limit himself to one or two slices of pizza without the crust and a small serving of ice cream. Feeling full, he may be able to skip the cake with frosting, the cookies, and the candy.

- When faced with the choice of healthy or happy, remember that healthy *is* happy. Do not give in every time your child plays on your heartstrings. Rather than respond impulsively, plan with your child when she can have desserts or special treats. Anticipation helps to satisfy a sweet tooth.

- Unless your child's blood sugars are very low, you can substitute honey or maple syrup for glucose tabs and avoid artificial flavoring and coloring.

- When making dietary changes, continually re-evaluate what you can handle. Take a step back if you are pushing yourself to the point of exhaustion.

- Stevia, a plant that is dried and ground to produce a sweet white powder, can be used as a sweetener to reduce your use of artificial sweeteners.

- Place a snack plate of green pepper, carrots, cucumbers, celery filled with peanut butter, and some ranch dressing next to your children when they are watching television, playing computer, or doing homework.

- Over time, add pieces of raw broccoli, cauliflower, baby tomatoes, red peppers, snap peas, green beans, or celery filled with almond butter or cream cheese. You can add chunks of cheese, rolled-up cold cuts, or fruit as well.

- A salad at dinner gives everyone raw, enzyme-rich food. Serve it before the meal when your children are really hungry.

- Suggestions for breakfast:

  Plain yogurt with a small amount of granola, frozen blueberries or sliced banana, and maple syrup or Stevia.

  Sprouted wheat toast or sprouted cinnamon toast with soy cream cheese and some fresh fruit.

  Fruit shakes made from bananas, milk, and any of the following: frozen blueberries, strawberries, raspberries, peaches, pineapple, or mango slices. You can sneak in plain yogurt or tofu for protein and add unsweetened cocoa for variety.

- Whole-grain bread French toast with fresh fruit and whipped cream.

- Suggested drinks to offer in place of juice:
  Hot cocoa: whole milk, unsweetened cocoa, one-half packet Stevia
  Lemonade: lemon juice, water, one-half packet Stevia
  Spritzer: seltzer, unsweetened cranberry juice, lime juice, one-half packet Stevia
  Hot vanilla milk: whole milk, cinnamon, vanilla, one-half packet Stevia

- For additional recipes go to www.challengeofdiabetes.com.

- As soon as possible, get your children used to drinking water with meals.

- As kids lower their sugar consumption, they crave less sweets.

- To develop a taste for healthy bread, move slowly from white bread to oat bran to whole wheat, and finally to a sprouted grain, such as Ezekiel. You can disguise whole grain bread as French toast or use it in grilled cheese sandwiches.

- Lettuce varies in nutritional value. Find dressing without sugar or corn syrup that your child likes and then move from iceberg lettuce to romaine and then to darker greens, such as red leaf lettuce or spinach.

- Keep a food log periodically, so that you know what your child is eating. You will be able to look back and see your progress over time.

Our Four-day Food Log After Diagnosis

Day	Breakfast	Snack	Lunch	2:30 Snack	4:00 Snack	Dinner	PM Snack
Carbs /meal total/day 335-350	75	30	60	20	40	80	30-45 depending on blood sugar #
Thursday	large bagel with butter 1 c. protein shake	1/2 5" cantaloupe 1 cup milk	German pancake roasted almonds applesauce milk	pineapple sugar-free Jell-O water	milk roasted almonds	1 chicken breast 1 & 1/2 cups noodles with butter	popcorn 8 pretzels milk
Friday	large bagel with butter 1 c. protein shake	popcorn	2 slices pizza cookie	apple	1/2 c. ice cream 1 c. milk	6 pieces sushi ribs	popcorn milk
Saturday	5 pancakes sugar-free syrup	banana cantaloupe	1 & 1/2 grilled cheese on white bread milk red pepper	apple	3/4 c. pretzel mix	German pancake snack mix carrots/ cucumber milk	white bread & butter milk
Sunday	4 pancakes sugar-free syrup milk	snack mix	1 & 1/2 grilled cheese on white bread milk red pepper/carrots	bag of Doritos	2 oz. cornbread protein shake	2 c. noodles with butter & parmesan cheese	cantaloupe milk

Two-year Food Log

Day	Breakfast	AM Snack	Lunch	2:30 Snack	4:00 Snack	Dinner	PM Snack
Carbs / meal 165-200	40-50	30	40	15	30	10-20	0-15 depending on blood sugar #
Monday	plain yogurt frozen blueberries homemade granola cut-up cantaloupe	almonds natural applesauce	peanut butter & jelly sandwich on oat-bran bread popcorn	orange slices cheese stick	snack plate of celery & peanut butter, cucumber, carrots, & apples	meatballs with sauce broccoli salad	blueberries & whipped cream
Tuesday	fruit smoothie sliced pear	almond cookies strawberries	turkey and cheese sandwich on oat bran bread carrots, & hummus	apple	homemade popsicle slice of sprouted bread with butter	vegetable soup cut vegetables	cheddar cheese slices
Wednesday	multigrain cereal milk banana	orange slices almonds	plain yogurt with granola popcorn celery with peanut butter	apple	turkey & cheese slices with chunks of melon	Thai food: vegetable soup chicken sate	almonds
Thursday	2 slices cinnamon & raisin sprouted bread with butter 3 chicken sausages apple slices	cantaloupe peanuts	Caesar salad with parmesan cheese chips & salsa	apple almonds	homemade ginger snaps with milk	chicken stir-fry salad	carrots & hummus
Friday	pancakes & bacon sugar-free syrup sugar-free hot cocoa	cheese puffs cashews	2 slices school pizza cut vegetables	orange cheese stick	Caesar salad apples almond butter	steak tips broccoli cut veggies	celery & peanut butter

Three-year Food Log

Day	Breakfast	AM Snack	Lunch	2:30 Snack	4:00 Snack	Dinner	PM Snack
Carbs /meal total/day 140-220	30-40	20-35	25-45	20-25	20-30	25-35	0-10 depending on blood sugar #
Thursday	plain yogurt with blueberries, homemade granola, & maple syrup	apple almond cookies	school salad bar with fruit salad glass of milk	energy bar with almonds, pecans, dates, cinnamon, cloves	lemonade (lemon juice, Stevia, water) cut veggies with hummus	roast chicken with broccoli & salad	banana slices with almond butter
Friday	French toast with whole grain bread, sugar-free syrup, bacon	popcorn orange	2 slices pizza (without crust) school salad bar & milk	apple	ice cream— frozen bananas, blackberries & coconut milk in blender	steak tips squash salad	raw whole milk
Saturday	cantaloupe slices cinnamon sprouted grain toast with butter	granola bar cheese	1 & 1/2 grilled cheese on sprouted wheat bread red pepper	grapes roasted cashews	banana with peanut butter seltzer with cherry juice, & Stevia	quesadillas on low-carb wraps cut vegetables with ranch dressing	nothing
Sunday	breakfast shake with banana, frozen berries, raw milk, & unsweetened cocoa	apple with almond butter	chicken Caesar salad sugar-free soda	granola bar	blueberries & whipped cream almond cookie	chicken kabobs stir-fry salad	nothing

- Quiet unobtrusive persistence usually wins out. Just as you are about to give up, your child will probably give in.

Sources of Information

- Read widely in large bookstores and public libraries.

- The American Diabetes Association has an outstanding list of practical guides on their Web site, diabetes.org.

- You can find Internet newsletters, research findings, and links to chat rooms from the following Web sites:
    childrenwithdiabetes.com
    diabetesincontrol.com
    enewsletter@jdrf.org(JDRF)

- *Dr. Bernstein's Diabetes Solution* by Richard K. Bernstein, M.D., is the most enlightening and important, albeit daunting, of all the books I read. The author, who has diabetes, explains why it is critically important to limit carbohydrates and get blood sugar numbers under control as soon as possible.

- Attend a Juvenile Diabetes Research Foundation coffee. Meetings usually feature a speaker, time for informal discussion, information, and networking opportunities.

- Read *Countdown to a Cure*, the quarterly magazine from the Juvenile Diabetes Research Foundation, which covers new developments in technology.

- Get information about complementary or holistic treatments. These healing modalities can be a very important addition to standard medical care.

- When trying any new supplements or treatments, set time limits and devise measurements. The better you measure the effects of a new variable, the sooner you can eliminate treatments that are not helping and feel confident about the ones that are.

Glossary of Terms

Acidophilus	A bacteria that foments milk and which is used to alter the bacterial flora in the gastrointestinal tract to treat certain digestive disorders.
Acupressure	An Eastern technique by which pressure is put on specific points of the body to realign the body's energy paths.
Acupuncture	An Eastern technique in which needles are inserted into specific points of the body in order to realign the energy paths and thus heal the body or relieve pain.
Adrenaline	A stress hormone from the adrenal glands that raises blood sugar levels.
Alpha cells	Cells in the pancreas that make glucagon.
Autoimmune disease	An illness through which the body's defense system attacks its own cells.
Beta cells	Cells in the pancreas that make and store insulin and release it into the bloodstream.
Bolus	An insulin injection to prevent the rise of blood sugar levels from a meal or to lower an already high blood sugar level.
Carbohydrate	One of the three basic sources of energy found in food; the others are protein and fat. A carbohydrate is a chain of sugar molecules such as cane, beet and grape sugar, starch, cellulose, and syrup.
Complex carbohydrate	A long chain of sugars which tends to be digested at a slower pace than simple carbohydrates.

C-peptide	"Connecting-peptide." A protein produced as a by-product of insulin. It is measured to estimate the insulin production of the pancreas.
Endocrine system	The system of glands and the hormones secreted by them. The endocrine glands are pituitary gland, thyroid, thymus, adrenal gland, pancreas, ovaries, and testes.
Glucagon	A hormone made by the alpha cells in the pancreas. It raises blood sugar levels by breaking down proteins and stored glycogen to glucose.
Glucose	A naturally occurring sugar. It is a building block of most carbohydrates and glycogen.
Glycemic index	A table which compares carbohydrates and foods according to how much they raise blood sugars.
Glycogen	A substance formed from glucose that is stored in the liver and muscles and can be quickly converted back to glucose.
Hemoglobin A1c	A blood test that measures how much glucose is bound to red blood cells. It indicates the average blood sugar level during a period of two to three months.
Honeymoon period	The period of remission after the original diagnosis of diabetes during which the pancreas resumes the production of some insulin.
Humalog	A brand of fast-acting insulin.
Hyperglycemia	Abnormally high blood sugar level.
Hypoglycemia	Abnormally low blood sugar level.
Immune system	The system which defends the body against foreign substances, such as bacteria and virus.
Insulin	A hormone produced by the pancreas' beta cells that helps glucose to enter the body's cells and thus provide them with energy.

Islets	A cluster of cells in the pancreas that includes alpha cells, which makes glucagon, and beta cells which make insulin. Also called the islets of Langerhans.
Juvenile diabetes	Diabetes that occurs in children and adolescents. This can be due to the destruction of insulin production (Type 1) or due to a developing resistance to insulin (Type 2).
Ketoacidosis	A condition in which the blood turns acidic, due to the presence of ketones in the bloodstream. This can cause a diabetic coma.
Ketones	Ketones are created when cells do not get enough energy due to a lack of insulin. Fat is then broken down into fatty acids and turns into ketones in the liver. The presence of ketones indicates that the blood sugar level is high.
Lantus	A long-acting form of insulin.
Metabolism	The complex chemical and physical processes that occur within a living cell or organism, which provide the energy and substances that are necessary to maintain life.
Pancreas	An abdominal organ which produces digestive enzymes and hormones, such as insulin and glucagon.
Spiking	An abrupt rise in the blood sugar level.
Stevia	A dried herb which is ground to produce a sweet-tasting white powder.
Ultralente	A long-acting form of insulin.

978-0-595-38625-3
0-595-38625-3